PRENATAL BOOKS FOR EXPECTING MOTHER

pregnancy, delivery, and newborn handbook.

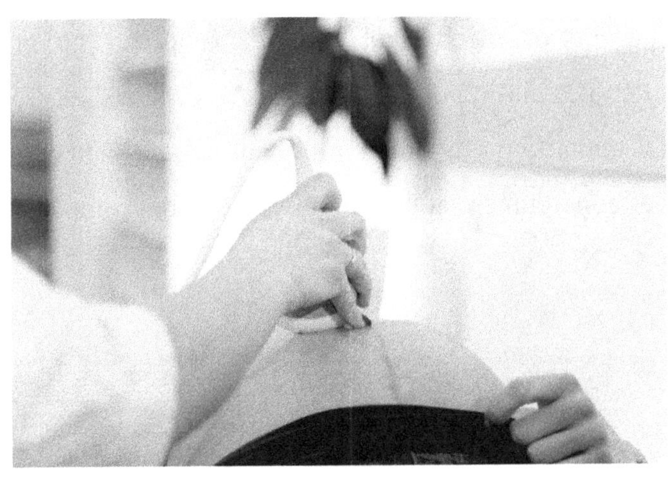

Ashley R.Whitlow

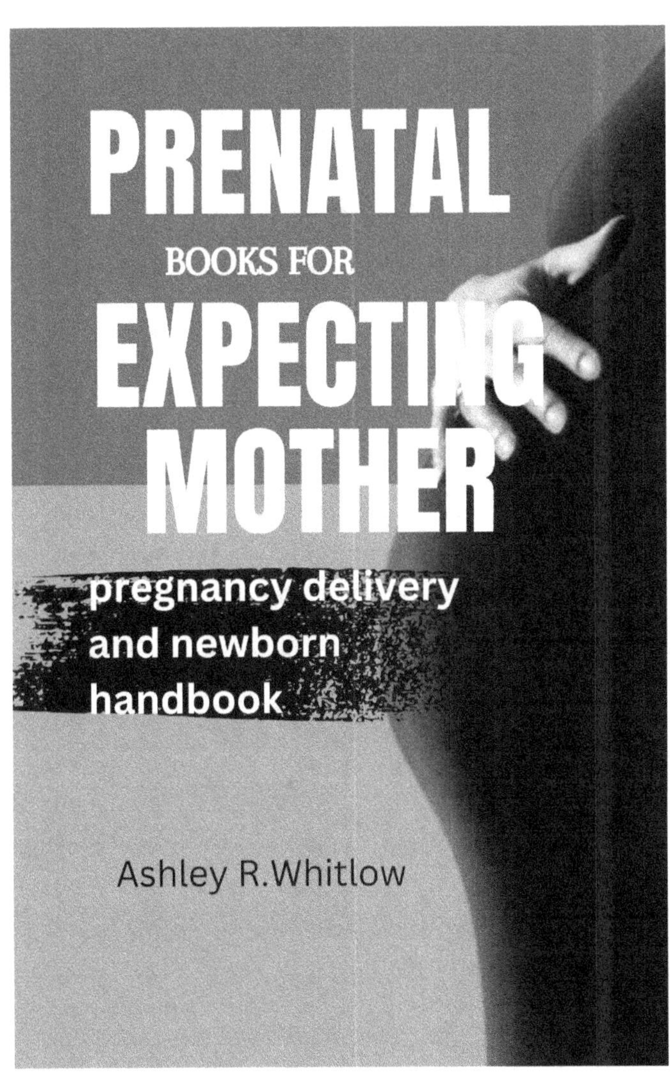

PRENATAL
BOOKS FOR
EXPECTING
MOTHER
pregnancy delivery
and newborn
handbook
Ashley R.Whitlow

TABLE OF CONTENT

Introduction: What to know ahead of being Pregnant

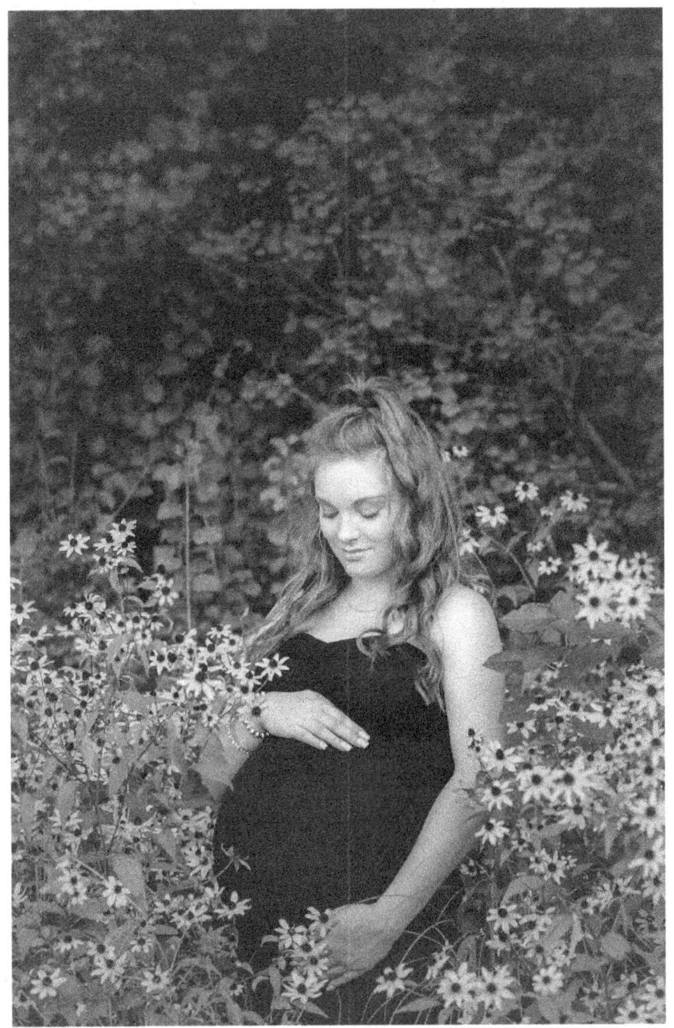

Congratulations on this incredible journey into motherhood! As you embark on the transformative adventure of pregnancy, this book is designed to be your trusted companion, providing guidance, support, and a wealth of information tailored to the unique experience of expecting mothers. From navigating the physical changes in your body to nurturing your emotional well-being, we aim to empower you with knowledge and insights that will enhance your prenatal journey. Get ready to embrace the joys, challenges, and the profound beauty of this miraculous time. This book is here to celebrate and support you every step of the way.

For many first-time moms, pregnancy is a combination of exuberant joy and overwhelming fear. The reason? Although a woman's pregnancy is a great and magnificent milestone in her life, numerous physical, hormonal, and psychological changes take place during this time, as well as the need to calm concerns and minimize stress. The following words of wisdom for prospective new moms stress the significance of the mind and body working in harmony to create the finest experience possible:

Counseling Before Pregnancy

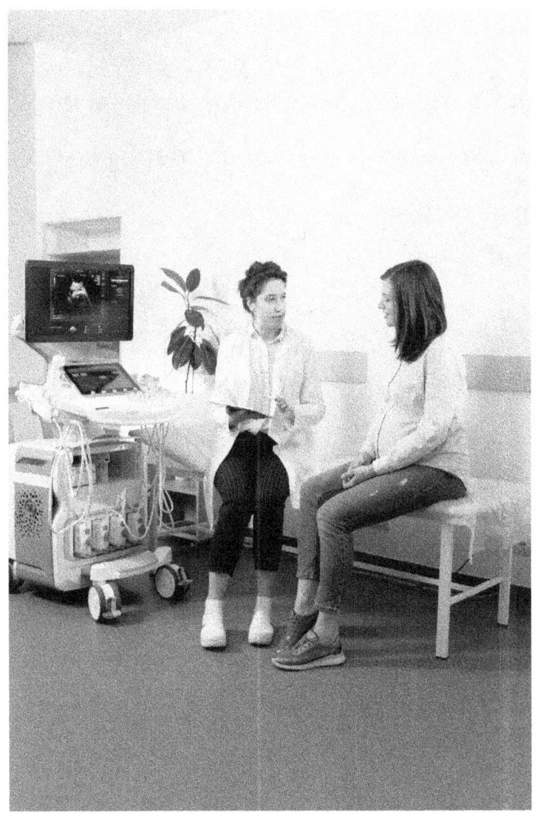

When you're prepared to start a family or grow it, make an appointment with your doctor or midwife for preconception counseling. Even if you've previously given birth, your provider may still examine you and determine if any new dangers need attention. Three months before you start trying to conceive, you should seek preconception counseling.

Your healthcare provider will talk about some aspects of your and your partner's health during preconception counseling, such as:

Personal medical history: Be sure to inform your doctor of any allergies, diabetes, high blood pressure, high blood sugar, epilepsy, or other conditions that might affect your pregnancy. It's important to have certain medical conditions under control before trying conception. Tell your doctor about all of your current medications, recent surgeries, and prior pregnancies, especially if you've had pregnancy complications like a loss.

A check of the mother and father's medical history may help determine whether either of them has ever had a condition that might be passed on to your child. If any members of your family have high blood pressure, diabetes, birth defects, intellectual disability, or any other health conditions, let your doctor know.

Several genetic disorders: This may be inherited (passed from parents to their children). Examples include sickle cell anemia, Tay-Sachs disease, and cystic fibrosis. The genes responsible for several genetic diseases may be found by blood tests done before pregnancy. Talk to your doctor about genetic testing before trying pregnancy.

Doctor verification: Your doctor will verify that you are up to date on all immunizations, including those for varicella and rubella (German measles), and will check your vaccination status (chickenpox). Pregnancy is not a safe time to get these immunizations, and being sick while expecting might cause miscarriage or malformed babies. Become the injections at least a month before trying to get pregnant if you don't already have immunity. You should also keep getting your annual flu vaccination, which is safe to get during all three trimesters of pregnancy.

Intimate partner violence (IPV) screening: Whether it be physical, sexual, or emotional abuse, intimate partner violence (IPV) refers to the abuse of a current or past spouse or partner. Coercion during pregnancy and throughout the reproductive process are also possibilities. The American College of Obstetricians and Gynecologists advises everyone who is thinking about becoming pregnant to be tested for IPV.

Prenatal examination: As part of preconception counseling, your doctor could advise getting health screening tests. A pre-pregnancy physical may involve the following:

I. Blood testing to establish your blood type and validate that you are STD-free.

II. A pelvic examination to look at your reproductive system's health (vagina, cervix, uterus, and ovaries).

III. A sample of the cells from your cervix is used in the Pap smear test to check for cancer.

IV. A physical examination checks your heart rate, blood pressure, pulse, and body temperature.

How To Prepare Your Body For Pregnancy

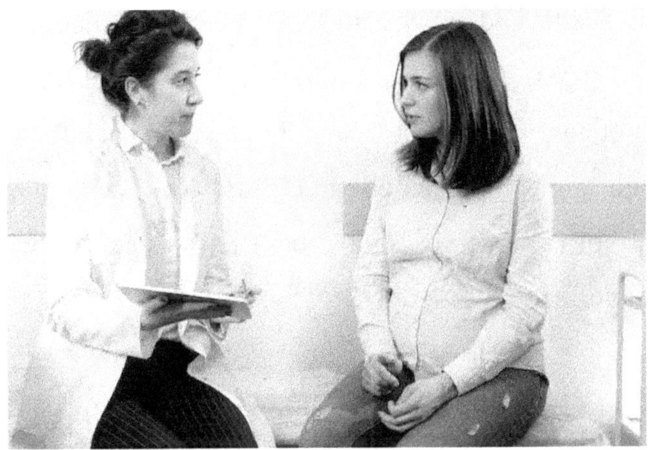

By preparing your body for pregnancy, you may guarantee that your health is at its best before becoming pregnant.

Abstain from alcohol: Drinking alcohol while attempting to conceive might harm your fertility. Ovulation, hormone levels, and your menstrual cycle all could be affected. Drinking while expecting may have serious consequences for the baby, including early birth and developmental delays.

Maintain a healthy diet: Eating a balanced diet is vital before and throughout pregnancy for both your overall health and the nutrition of the baby. Choose a range of fruits, vegetables, healthy grains, low-fat dairy, lean proteins, and low-fat dairy products. Avoid foods that are highly processed and fatty. The maximum quantity of caffeine you should have daily is one to two cups of coffee.

Preventing exposure to harmful substances: Pregnant women should refrain from exposure to radiation, toxic chemicals (like lead), and pesticides. The developing foetus may be negatively impacted by exposure to high doses of various radiation types, as well as some chemicals and dangerous substances.

Exercise often and maintain a healthy weight: Being active and maintaining a healthy weight are essential before and throughout pregnancy. Women who are overweight are more likely to acquire diabetes and high blood pressure. Low birth weights are possible in children born to underweight moms.

Recognize domestic violence: Women who have been subjected to abuse in the past may be more likely to suffer it now that they are expecting a child. Asking your doctor or a midwife for support may help you find the community, social, and legal support you need to deal with domestic violence.

Give up smoking: Studies show that babies delivered to smoker mothers are more likely to be premature, have smaller birth weights, and have sudden infant death syndrome (SIDS). Furthermore, moms who are exposed to secondhand smoke are more likely to have underweight children. The chemicals, particles, and gases left behind after smoking tobacco and found on clothing, furniture, and hair, also known as thirdhand smoke, may be hazardous.

Be caution: To lower your chance of becoming sick, stay away from undercooked meat and raw eggs. Additionally, avoid touching or coming in contact with animal excrement, cat litter, or any other materials that might potentially contain harmful parasites or viruses. Keep your distance from sick people and wash your hands often.

Start taking vitamins: Start taking a prenatal vitamin or a daily vitamin with 400 mcg of folic acid. Folic acid consumption may reduce the chance of neural tube abnormalities, which are birth deformities of the brain and spinal cord.

Fill Nutritional Gaps in Your Diet by Taking a Prenatal Vitamin *Everyday* Because they assist in completing any nutritional gaps that may occur in your diet, prenatal vitamins are crucial throughout pregnancy.

Consider taking an omega-3 supplement throughout pregnancy that is devoid of mercury to help with depressive symptoms. The nutrients and minerals in prenatal vitamins are vital for the development of your unborn child. They include calcium, iron, iodine, and folic acid.

Did you know that it's recommended to take a prenatal vitamin every day while trying to become pregnant to help your baby grow better during the first month of pregnancy when the brain and spinal cord form? The fact that many would-be dads are ignorant of the need for dietary folic acid, zinc, and vitamin C for healthy sperm development and quality is also notable.

Follow the birth plan you decide on: Early on in your pregnancy, decide what sort of birth you want to have, and then take steps to increase your chances of obtaining it. This comprises creating the birth plan you choose, including specifics such as your decision to use or refrain from taking medicines throughout labor and delivery. You may consider destroying the plan now that you've written it down and have an idea since labor is full of surprises and having a strategy can make it tougher for you to roll with the punches.

Participate in Prenatal Yoga Classes and Keep Up Your Exercise Routine: Yoga is a great method to stay fit, active, and calm down when pregnant. The focus of this kind of yoga, which was created particularly for expecting moms, is on poses that increase flexibility and strength. Expectant women may benefit from prenatal yoga by preserving their physical and mental wellness. It also offers breathing exercises and relaxation techniques to help with labor.

Exercise during pregnancy does reduce the incidence of gestational diabetes, enhances and maintains fitness, and aids in weight management. Women who are expecting should never exercise without first getting approval from their doctor. It is recommended that pregnant women do

150 minutes of weekly moderate-intensity aerobic activity.

The 150 minutes may be divided into daily exercises of 10 minutes or lengthier workouts of 30 minutes on five days of the week. Walking, jogging, biking, utilizing a rowing machine, an elliptical machine, or swimming are a few strategies to enhance energy output. Women who have never worked out while pregnant should begin slowly and gradually raise their activity level; those who have worked out in the past should keep working out as long as their doctor gives the all-clear.

Pass the PreTRM examination: PreTRM, a brand-new blood test, may tell if a pregnant woman is at risk of delivering birth too soon. A protein that predicts a preterm birth in the 19th or 20th week of pregnancy is looked for in the blood. Those women who should pay special attention to this exam are:

IVF treatments were performed or pregnancy-related medical attention was needed having problems becoming pregnant, choosing to have a baby after reaching 35, and having already had a miscarriage.

Sign up for a support group: By joining a support group, first-time expectant women may strengthen their relationships with their families, friends, and other mothers. Women may discuss pertinent topics and share parenting advice in a safe setting provided by support groups. The pregnant mother builds a strong network of lasting ties by making new connections with others going through similar experiences.

Question your physician: Throughout your pregnancy, it is essential to address any concerns and symptoms with your doctor, even the uncomfortable ones. Do not immediately go online and begin searchingly for answers to your concerns (it is very common for unpleasant and odd symptoms to develop). Instead, schedule a consultation with your doctor and list your concerns in writing so you won't forget them. My motto is "do not confuse my medical degree with your Google search."

Keep an eye on your weight gain: Women who are expecting should monitor their weight to make sure they don't put on too little or too much. She should regularly monitor her weight on her own and speak with her doctor if it rises. It's crucial to understand that a woman who had a healthy weight before becoming pregnant often gained 25 to 35 pounds throughout her pregnancy.

Have a good time: As a prospective mother who will bring another human into the world, you are a superhero. Keep in mind that even superheroes need rest. The occasional, safe indulgence is essential to a good and pleasant pregnancy. In other words, do some investigating.

This may be as simple as getting some sleep or taking a warm bath, getting a prenatal massage, practicing meditation for five minutes every day, or going to a yoga class to reduce stress.

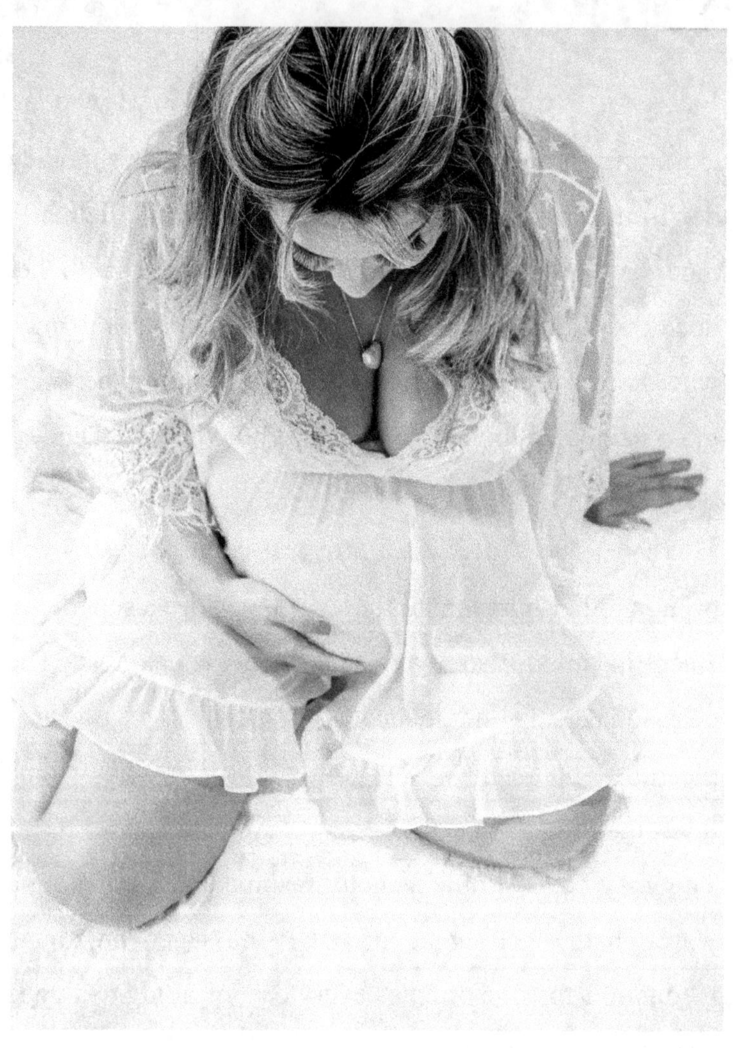

Chapter 1: Needs of a newly pregnant mom

Even though being pregnant is lovely and magical, there are many side effects, aches and pains, and unsolved concerns that come with it. Additionally, all of a sudden, your clothing stop fitting. When you are pregnant, there are a few necessities that will make the process healthier and more pleasant. The lengthy list of pregnant necessities, though, may sometimes feel a bit overwhelming.

The fact is that you don't need much more to have a baby than a balanced diet and frequent doctor's appointments.

You only have the baby for nine months, so you don't want to spend excessively or store up. Nevertheless, there are a few inexpensive goods that might make it a bit easier for you to get through your pregnancy.

Vitamins for pregnancy. Prenatal vitamins are recommended for all pregnant women, even though it is possible to survive pregnancy without taking them. This is because it might be challenging to receive all the nourishment you need from diet alone.

You need more vitamins and minerals, such as folic acid, iron, and calcium, during pregnancy. Additionally, a lot of us struggle to consume a balanced diet when we experience food intolerances or morning sickness.

You'll probably get a prescription for prenatal vitamins from your doctor. Some women may handle them well, but many find that when they have morning sickness, they are difficult to swallow or digest. Most medical professionals will work with you to compare prenatal until you discover one that you like.

It's best to avoid purchasing a lot of prenatal vitamins at once, particularly in the first trimester, since your preferences may change. But it also works if you discover a prenatal vitamin that you like and want to buy plenty of. You should plan to incorporate prenatal vitamins into your budget for quite some time if you want to breastfeed since you will need to continue taking your prenatal vitamins while doing so.

Morning sickness and gastrointestinal treatments. Almost everyone experiences a bit of nauseated throughout the first trimester of pregnancy, and even beyond that, whether or not they vomit while pregnant. Things like constipation and heartburn then start to appear as the pregnancy goes on.

Although it's impossible to forecast which of these conditions you'll experience and when you may wish to buy a few things to make yourself more comfortable at some point throughout your pregnancy.

Anti-nausea wristbands, morning sickness lollipops, teas, plain crackers, and pretzels are all common morning sickness remedies.
For the safe medication to treat heartburn and constipation, see your doctor. The majority of

over-the-counter medicines are efficient and safe to use in treating these symptoms while pregnant.

It's not essential to buy every product on the market at once if you end up experiencing morning sickness or digestive issues. You may give one or two choices a trial before continuing. Even while dealing with these issues while they are occurring is bothersome, they often go away on their own.

A Reliable Moisturizer. You may notice certain skin changes as your tummy stretches and expands. Dry, itchy skin is typical. Additional dry skin on your face and elsewhere may also be a problem. As their skin expands, a lot of women get stretch marks on their bellies. 6 Be aware that there is little proof that over-the-counter treatments for stretch marks are effective.

In any case, moisturizing your stomach and other dry skin spots may be quite relaxing and can help relieve any itching. The majority of straightforward, over-the-counter moisturizers are safe for expectant mothers, but you may inquire with your doctor about any specific compounds you should avoid.

For instance, it is often not advised for pregnant women to use additives like retinoids, retinol, hydroquinone, benzoyl peroxide, and salicylic acid. A moisturizer that is as natural and chemical-free as possible is often the best option.

Keep a bottle of your favorite moisturizer in your medicine cabinet or beside your bed for daily use after you've discovered one you enjoy. Applying it to your expanding tummy may be soothing and a fantastic opportunity to unwind and develop a relationship with the baby within.

Abdominal support band Back discomfort, sacroiliac (SI) joint pain, and hip and abdominal aches are all typical as your belly expands and your center of gravity changes. Wearing a belt or belly band that is supportive helps many ladies. These elastic bands support your back while also preventing your tummy from dropping.

When your belly becomes big and noticeable, generally at the end of the second trimester or the start of the third, belly support bands are often utilized. They are particularly beneficial for expectant mothers who wish to stay active or who may be more susceptible to muscular injuries associated with pregnancy.

During pregnancy, a single belly support band is all that is required. Considering that not all women find them useful, it is better to hold off on buying one until you are big enough to truly need one. Since their bodies are recuperating throughout the postpartum time, many women choose to keep wearing their bands. The majority of belly bands are affordable and may be worn again during a second pregnancy.

In-body pillow. It might be challenging to find a sleeping posture that is comfortable as your tummy grows. As your belly swells, you shouldn't sleep on your back because you run the danger of narrowing the arteries and blood vessels that provide your unborn child with oxygen. The more your belly grows, sleeping on your stomach becomes a clear challenge. During the second and third trimesters, side sleeping is recommended, although even that may become painful.

the pregnant body pillow comes in. These pillows may be wonderful for expecting mothers since they provide additional support for your hips, back, and legs as you find the most comfortable side-lying position—which is the recommended sleeping posture throughout pregnancy. They may also relieve joint pressure. A cushion is often positioned between the legs of women to realign the hip joints and relieve strain.

There are several forms, sizes, materials, and softness/firmness options for pregnancy pillows. It's advisable to visit a shop to test out a few. Most likely, you'll only need one when pregnant. You may put it away after giving birth, but if you're very connected to yours, you could continue to use it for months thereafter. You can even use it for future pregnancies.

Bra that supports. Your breasts will enlarge by at least one cup size when you're pregnant, and they'll also become heavier and uncomfortable, particularly in the first trimester. You'll probably need a new bra at least once while you're pregnant. As your breasts will continue to expand during your pregnancy, choose one that is supportive, gentle, and adaptable.

If you want to nurse, you could think about purchasing a nursing bra (with latches on the cups for simple opening) and wearing it during your pregnancy. However, if you want to start using a nursing bra while you are pregnant, be aware that breastfeeding will cause your breasts to become even larger.

When your breasts start to expand in preparation for nursing during the first trimester, you'll probably need to start using a larger bra. You may need to buy two or three new bras, depending on how often you wash your bras in general and if you require a sports bra or another specialized kind.

Maternity Apparel. For the majority of us, buying maternity clothing is a no-brainer. After all, when you are pregnant, you will eventually outgrow your ordinary clothing. 13 A positive pregnancy test might cause some individuals to be unable to fasten their trousers as soon as a few days afterward.

Maternity pants are probably the thing you'll need to stock up on the most, but you may get away with a waist expander or simply some comfy sweatpants for a time. As your belly, waistline, rib cage, and breasts expand and increase during the second trimester, you will require maternity shirts and trousers.
You don't need to purchase any particular footwear, but as the months go by, your feet may enlarge and swell, making heels unappealing to wear often.

When you are expecting, it might be tempting to purchase a whole new outfit, but it is not essential. A week's worth of tops and bottoms, along with a couple of new, larger bras, is all you need if you want to keep to the fundamentals. As you shop, bear in mind that you'll probably continue to wear your maternity pants after your baby is delivered, so it makes sense to spend money on a few goods, comfortable ones.

Maternity books. Each week of your pregnancy will be distinct from the one before it, and both your body and your unborn child will develop and change in several novel and fascinating ways. But on occasion, the situation might be perplexing and upsetting, and it's normal to wonder what is happening to your body.

As the month's pass, a good pregnancy book—especially one with images and illustrations—can serve as a dependable pregnant companion. Most books will assist you in getting ready for your prenatal checkups and will include advice on what to anticipate during birthing and afterward in addition to detailing fetal growth and physical changes associated with pregnancy.

You just need one or two novels that you adore and trust. Pregnancy books are often available at your local library or used bookstore. A smart approach is always to ask friends for suggestions. Pick a book that gives you a sense of comfort, isn't too clinical, and presents information in a comprehensive and balanced manner.

When you're having a baby, you concentrate a lot on what your baby will require, and purchasing small newborn apparel and accessories is a lot of fun. But expecting mothers also need to be catered to since they have unique demands. After all, albeit a joy, being pregnant can also be very physically and emotionally taxing.

A sleep, a lengthy bath, and the opportunity to put your feet up are maybe the nicest presents you can give yourself and don't even come with a price tag. Spending money on some R & R now is a smart move since it won't be available once the baby is born.

Keep it simple, but don't cut corners. You have the right to get whatever it is you need to make the next nine months as pleasant and comfortable as possible.

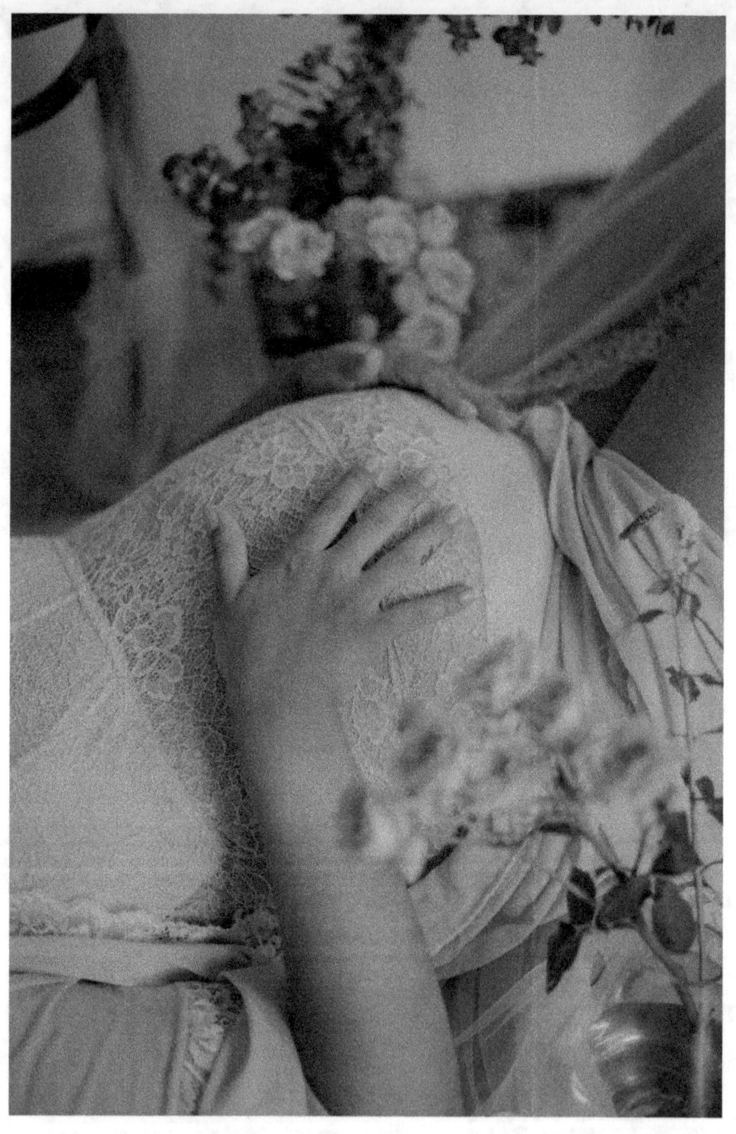

Chapter 2: What to expect during the first trimester of pregnancy and nutrition guide.

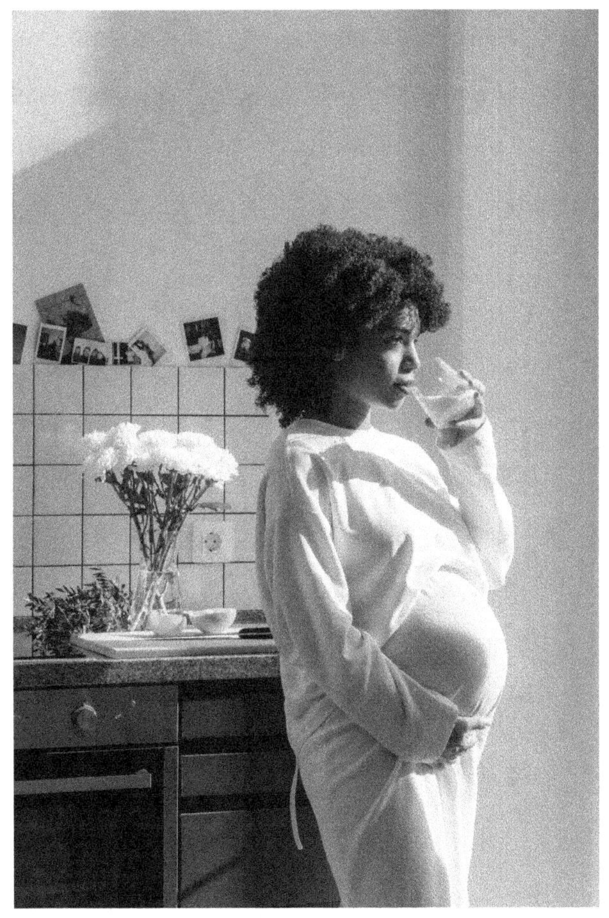

Greetings from the thrilling and life-changing world of pregnancy! An amazing journey full of mind-blowing transformations and an emotional rollercoaster begins during the first trimester. We delve into the unique aspects of the first three months in this book, providing insightful information on what to anticipate during this critical time. From the first indications of pregnancy to the peak of your child's growth, we are here to support you through every step of the journey.

Not only that, but diet is essential for maintaining your health and your baby's during this period of development. With the help of our in-depth nutritional guide, you'll be able to make educated decisions and guarantee that you get the necessary nutrients for a successful pregnancy. Equipped with knowledge and a guide for prospering throughout this extraordinary first trimester, let's go out on this amazing journey.

The First Trimester.

The first 12 weeks of pregnancy are a time of significant physical change for a woman. Women often begin to worry about:

Making educated choices and being ready for the significant changes that lie ahead are made easier when you understand a pregnancy week by week.

An average pregnancy lasts for 40 weeks. Three trimesters are formed from the weeks. The period from conception to week 12 of pregnancy is known as the first trimester.

What changes does the female body go through in the first trimester?

The first trimester is a time of significant physical change for women. The body produces hormones that have an impact on practically every organ. Missing your period is the first indication that you could be pregnant. Following the first few weeks, some women report the following:

Fatigue, nausea, diarrhea, mood changes, sore breasts, weight gain, headaches, food cravings, food aversions, and constipation.

During this period, you may need to sleep more or eat more often. However, some women have none of these symptoms at all.

What occurs to the developing fetus in the first trimester?

Your last menstrual cycle began on the first day of your pregnancy. An egg is released 10 to 14 days later, a sperm and an egg interact, and pregnancy takes place. During the first trimester, a baby grows quickly. The organs start to grow, and the brain and spinal cord start to develop in the fetus. The first trimester is also when the baby's heart starts to beat.

In the first few weeks, arms and legs start to bud, and by the end of eight weeks, fingers and toes start to take shape. The developing baby's sex organs are developed by the end of the first trimester.

What may one anticipate from the physician?

Make an appointment with your doctor as soon as you find out you are pregnant to start providing for the growing child. Start taking prenatal vitamins right away if you aren't already. Prenatal vitamins that include folic acid should be taken by women for a year before conception. In the first trimester, doctors often visit women once per month.

Your initial appointment will include a thorough health history questionnaire, a complete physical examination, and a pelvic exam. The physician might also conduct an ultrasound to verify pregnancy, do a Pap test, measuring your blood pressure, test for hepatitis, HIV, and sexually transmitted diseases.

Other tests may include calculate your due date, which is around 266 days from the start of your previous period check for danger signs like anemia, assess the thyroid levels, and check your weight.

The doctor will conduct a procedure known as nuchal translucency (NT) scan at around 11 weeks. The baby's head and neck are measured during the examination using an ultrasound. The measures may be used to calculate the likelihood that your child will have Down syndrome, a genetic condition. Consult your doctor to find out whether genetic testing is advised for your pregnancy. To determine your baby's risk for certain genetic illnesses, you may do a genetic screening test.

What can I do to maintain my health during the first trimester?

To take care of herself and her growing kid, a woman must be informed of what to do and what to avoid while pregnant.

Things to do

Following are some wise personal health precautions to make in the first trimester:

Prenatal vitamins are advised, as is frequent exercise.

By doing Kegel exercises, you may strengthen your pelvic floor.

Consume a diet rich in fiber, low-fat protein sources, fruits, and vegetables.

Get plenty of water.

Consume enough energy (about 300 calories more than normal).

What not to do

Avoiding the following throughout the first trimester:

Workout or strength training that is physically Demanding yet might harm your stomach.

Alcohol.

Caffeine (no more than one cup of coffee or tea per day).

Smoking and illicit substances.

Smoked fish or raw seafood (no sushi).

White snapper fish, sharks, swordfish, or mackerel (they have high levels of mercury).

Fresh sprouts.

Toxoplasmosis is a parasite illness that may be spread through cat litter.

Unpasteurized dairy products, such as milk.

What else has to be taken into account during the first trimester?

During the first trimester, there are many physical changes to consider, but having a baby will also have an impact on other aspects of your life. During the first few months of your pregnancy, you should start thinking about a lot of things so you can be ready for the future.

When should you inform your family, friends, and employer?

You may wish to hold off until the pregnancy enters the second trimester as the first trimester is when miscarriages are most likely.

As your pregnancy develops, you may want to think about continuing to work or quitting, as well as if your company offers unpaid maternity leave for childbirth and care.

Healthy Dietary Advice During The First Trimester.

Eating healthy may have slipped off your priority list during the first trimester of pregnancy due to morning sickness and heartburn.

Right now, your body is going through a hormonal surge that might make you feel sick. Progesterone in particular has been linked to digestive issues including indigestion and constipation.

Many expectant mothers discover during the early stages of pregnancy that they are unable to maintain their prior appetite for certain nutritious items, such as lean meats or fresh vegetables. (Don't be alarmed; many pregnant women regain their appetite in the second trimester.)

For the time being, don't stress out too much if you're not in the mood to fill your plate to the brim at every meal. Instead, concentrate on these healthy meals throughout the first trimester to meet all of your nutritional needs.

During the first trimester, how many more calories should you consume?

Your baby's energy requirements throughout the first trimester are much like your baby's! They are still really little. In the first trimester, you should try to consume about 2,000 calories each day, but your doctor could advise more depending on your level of activity. This figure is generally in line with guidelines for adult nutrition.

Try to consume three meals and one or two snacks each day. If you have problems controlling your portion sizes, focus on quality instead. Make sure the food you do manage to eat is both nourishing and enjoyable to you at the time. (We understand that throughout pregnancy, your appetite and tolerance levels might fluctuate hour by hour.)

Maintain your healthy eating habits and create a first-trimester diet that is nutritious.

Drinks For Pregnant Women in first trimester

Folic Acid. Regarding nutrition during the first trimester and prenatal nutrition in general, this is the most important vitamin. This is due to the important function that folic acid, commonly known as vitamin B9 or folate when it is found in the diet, plays in avoiding neural tube abnormalities. Take a daily prenatal vitamin and consume foods like oranges, strawberries, green leafy vegetables, fortified morning cereals, kidney beans, almonds, cauliflower, and beets to receive the 600 micrograms per day that are advised.

Protein. It is essential for the formation of uterine tissue and the development of muscles in both you and your unborn child. Per day, aim for roughly 75 grams. Greek yogurt, poultry, and eggs are all excellent sources.

Calcium. It's essential for the growth of your baby's bones and teeth. Too little calcium in your diet may eventually lead to brittle bones (osteoporosis) since your developing baby will use calcium from your reserves. A well-balanced diet that includes milk, cheese, yogurt, and dark leafy greens may usually provide you with the 1,000 milligrams per day that are advised, but if you're concerned that you may not be getting enough, ask your OB/GYN whether you should take a supplement.

Iron. As your blood supply rises to meet the needs of your developing baby, iron becomes more and more crucial. To lessen your chance of developing pregnant anemia, make sure you're receiving a good amount of iron in your prenatal vitamin as the recommended daily intake of 27 milligrams might be difficult to meet via food alone. Include healthy sources like spinach, steak, poultry, eggs, and tofu in your diet plan.

Oranges, broccoli, and strawberries are foods high in vitamin C, which helps your developing baby's bones and tissues develop and increases iron absorption. The daily target amount should be 85 milligrams.

Potassium. Together with salt, it helps your body maintain the right balance of fluids while also controlling blood pressure. Use your prenatal vitamin and fruits like bananas, apricots, and avocados to obtain 2,900 milligrams each day.

DHA. DHA, an essential omega-3 fatty acid, is present in fish low in mercury, such as anchovies, herring, and sardines. These days, you may feel too sick to eat seafood, so talk to your doctor about taking a DHA supplement.

Things to eat during your first trimester

The following foods are specifically recommended by nutritionists because they are abundant sources of the vitamins, minerals, and macronutrients that your body (and the growing body of your kid) need to flourish.

Fatty meat. Thoroughly cooked lean meats, such as sirloin or chuck steak, pork tenderloin, turkey, and chicken, provide all of the amino acids that serve as the building blocks for cells and are a rich source of iron and protein.

Yogurt. Each cup's protein and calcium help to maintain healthy bones. Choose a type with a limited number of ingredients and little added sugars.

Edamame. These soybean pods include a significant amount of vegetarian protein in addition to calcium, iron, and folate.

Kale. The combination platter of nutrients in this dark leafy green includes fiber, calcium, folate, iron, vitamin A, vitamin C, vitamin E, and vitamin K.

Bananas. Bananas are one of the finest nutritional sources of potassium and are bland enough to be edible for unsettled tummies.

lentils and beans. These little yet potent powerhouses include iron, folate, protein, and fiber.

ginger brew. Products containing ginger, such as ginger tea and ginger chews, may help treat nausea.

Eating advice if you have nausea and morning sickness?

During the first three months of pregnancy, over 75% of expectant mothers suffer nausea, stomachaches, or other morning sickness symptoms.

To reduce nausea:

Instead of forcing yourself to eat three substantial meals a day, fuel yourself with several little meals every few hours. Both going too long without eating and eating huge meals have the potential to exacerbate nausea.

Steer clear of spicy and very fatty meals since they might cause heartburn or stomach pain.

When you're feeling queasy, stick to cold or room-temperature bland meals, such as yogurt with fruit, string cheese with nuts, or a mini-baguette with nut butter. Hot meals are more likely to release smells that might worsen nausea.

Eat meals with fluids or a soft texture. When your stomach is unsettled, you may find it easier to tolerate a homemade smoothie, oatmeal, or noodles.

Keep dry, convenient snacks available, such as in your handbag or work bag as well as on your bedside. Pretzels, low-sugar dry cereal, and Graham crackers are excellent grab-and-go choices.

How to eat healthy during the first trimester

Throughout the end, it's crucial to eat healthily in the first trimester, but try not to obsess about what you're placing on your plate, as this may add needless stress to a period that is probably already rife with anxiety.

Although diversity is vital, once your nausea and morning sickness in the second trimester go away, you'll probably find it easier to load your plate with a larger variety of meals. Take it easy on yourself and your stomach for the time being. Do not overlook:

Remain hydrated. Before going to sleep, fill a glass with water and set it on your bedside. When you awake, sip from it before beginning the day. If you think plain water sounds bland, try adding a piece of lemon, a cucumber, or some fresh berries.

Snack wisely. Early in pregnancy, sudden hunger with accompanying nausea and even fullness are frequent symptoms. By having nutritious snacks throughout the day, such as a small handful of nuts, a few whole-grain crackers with cheese, a piece of fresh fruit, or a slice of whole-grain toast with nut butter, you may maintain a stable blood sugar level.

Prenatal, pop that. Everyone doesn't eat precisely every day, which is one of the reasons why taking prenatal vitamins is so crucial. Make a phone alarm to remind you to take your vitamin every day.

Consult your OB/GYN if you're unsure. He or she may provide you with advice on which foods and beverages, such as alcohol, unpasteurized dairy products, and undercooked meats, you should avoid during the first trimester.

How You Can Stop a Miscarriage

Genetic disorders in the developing fetus are the main reason for miscarriages. Sadly, there is little that can be done to stop miscarriages brought on by inherited defects.

However, not every miscarriage is brought on by a genetic anomaly. If you've experienced a miscarriage, see your doctor as soon as possible to try to pinpoint the cause and make plans for another pregnancy. Healthy habits may be beneficial both before and throughout pregnancy. The following advice might help women avoid miscarriages:

If feasible, start taking 400 mcg of folic acid every day at least one to two months before conception.

Regular exercise Eat nutritious, balanced meals.

Stress management. Be sure to maintain a healthy weight. Don't smoke.Don't use illegal substances and make sure your vaccines are current.

A miscarriage may be avoided by taking these precautions as well:

Avoid radiation and toxins including ethylene oxide, arsenic, lead, formaldehyde, and lead.

Take extra precautions to protect your abdomen when you are expecting. Avoid engaging in riskier activities like contact sports and skiing, and always buckle your seatbelt.

Before taking any medication, including over-the-counter medicines, while pregnant, see your healthcare professional.

Finding out about and taking care of any health issues you may have before trying for a baby will also assist to guarantee that your child is healthy. Consider seeking therapy for the underlying issue, such as if you are aware that a prior miscarriage was brought on by an immunological reaction or a hormone imbalance. To increase your chances of having a safe pregnancy after you get pregnant, seek out early, thorough prenatal care.

Chapter 3: The second trimester of pregnancy nutrition advice

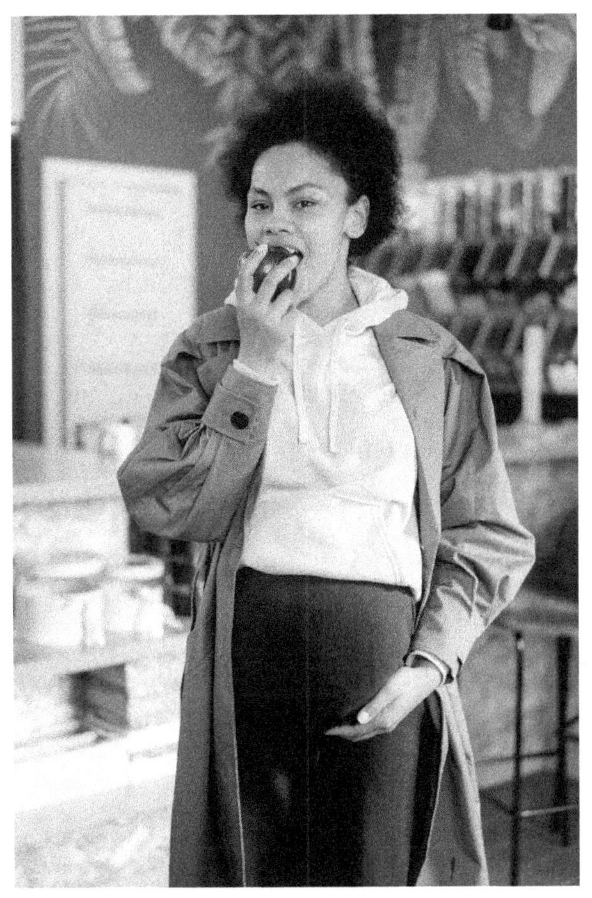

Your pregnancy's second trimester comprises weeks 13 to 28, or months 4, 5, and 6. During this stage of pregnancy, you can begin to see your "baby bump" and feel your unborn child move for the first time.

Your morning sickness and lethargy from the previous three months should subside as you start your second trimester of pregnancy.

For many women, the second three months of pregnancy are the most straightforward. When you are feeling better and have more energy, start making preparations for the birth of your child.

The second trimester is a time of rapid growth for your unborn child. You'll get an ultrasound between the 18th and 22nd week of pregnancy so your doctor can monitor the development of your unborn child. If you don't mind being shocked, you can also find out your baby's sex. Additionally, you can learn whether you are carrying twins during this trimester.

What to anticipate In Your Body during 3rd trimester

Your Lower Abdomen Feels achy. You can have some cramping or discomfort in your lower abdomen during the second trimester. The expansion of your uterus during pregnancy exerts strain on adjacent muscles and ligaments, which causes cramps. Your round ligament muscle often cramps as it expands throughout your second trimester.

In addition to a persistent soreness in your lower abdomen, you could also experience sudden acute pains. Minor cramps are common and might be brought on by intercourse, gas, or even constipation. Try taking a warm bath, using relaxation techniques, moving about, or applying a hot water bottle wrapped in a towel to your lower tummy to ease the pain.

Backache. Your back is beginning to feel achy and uncomfortable due to the additional weight you've added over the last several months. Use a chair with adequate back support and sit up straight to relieve the strain. With a cushion between your legs, lie on your side. Do not lift or carry anything heavy. Put on comfortable, low-heeled shoes with strong arch support. If the discomfort is severe, ask your spouse to massage the painful areas or treat yourself to a prenatal massage.

Gum bleeding. The majority of pregnant women have swollen sensitive gums. Your gums are becoming more sensitive and bleeding more often as a result of hormonal changes that are causing more blood to be sent to them. After the birth of your child, your gums ought to return to normal. Use a gentler toothbrush in the meantime, and be careful while flossing, but don't compromise on oral hygiene. According to studies, pregnant women with gum disease (also known as periodontal disease) may be more likely to have early labor and give birth to an underweight baby.

Contractions that are Braxton-Hicks. During the second trimester, you can begin to feel your uterus' muscles tighten for a minute or two. These symptoms are not actual contractions or other symptoms of labor. They could appear and disappear at random, and their rhythm and power can be erratic. More often than not, these muscular spasms are more uncomfortable than painful.

Braxton-Hicks contractions may be brought on by sex, strenuous activity, dehydration, a full bladder, or even by someone touching your growing baby. During these contractions, you may practice your labor breathing methods. Take a warm bath, have a cup of herbal tea, alter your posture, or increase your water intake to help you relax.

Expansion of the breasts. Although most of the breast soreness you had in the first trimester should have subsided, your breasts are still expanding in preparation for feeding your baby. You may feel more at ease by wearing a decent support bra and going up one or more bra sizes.

Nosebleeds and congestion. The mucus membranes lining your nose enlarge as a result of hormonal changes, which may produce a stuffy nose and cause you to snore at night. Your nose may bleed more often as a result of these changes. Consult your doctor before taking a decongestant.

There may be safer alternatives to treat congestion during pregnancy, such as saline drops and other natural remedies. To maintain moisture in the air, you may also consider using a humidifier. Maintaining a straight posture with your head up and not tilted back can help you stop bleeding from the nose by applying pressure to the nostril for a few minutes.

Discharge. Early in your pregnancy, you may have leukorrhea, a thin, milky white vaginal discharge that is typical. If it helps you feel more at ease, you may use a panty liner. However, avoid using tampons since they might contaminate the vagina. Call your doctor if the discharge smells bad, is green or yellow, bloody, or if there is a lot of clear discharge.

Dizziness. During the second trimester, as your uterus grows, it pushes on blood arteries, which sometimes makes you feel lightheaded. Low blood sugar levels and pregnancy-related hormone changes are other factors. Don't remain still for too long. Sit up gently or get out of bed. Frequently consume meals and snacks. Remain hydrated. Throughout the remainder of your pregnancy, avoid taking hot baths or showers and wear loose clothing. If you have dizziness or fainting, as well as vaginal bleeding or stomach discomfort, call your doctor right once.

A lot of urine. During the second trimester, your uterus will separate from the pelvic cavity, offering you a temporary respite from needing to often use the restroom. But don't settle in too much. During your last trimester of pregnancy, the need to relieve yourself will return.

Hair expansion hormones. Hair expansion Hormones related to pregnancy may speed up hair growth, but not necessarily in the desired places. Your hair on top of your head will thicken. Additionally, you can see hair growing in unexpected areas including your cheeks, arms, and back. Although they may not be the simplest solutions, shaving and tweezing are your best choices at this time. Because there is still more study to be done, many specialists advise against using depilatories, electrolysis, waxing, or laser hair removal while pregnant. Hear what your doctor advises by asking.

Headache. One of the most typical pregnancy concerns is a headache. Get lots of sleep, and work on relaxing exercises like deep breathing. Ibuprofen and aspirin are contraindicated during pregnancy, but if you're genuinely in pain, your doctor could allow you to take acetaminophen.

 These are brought on by your body producing more progesterone, a hormone. The muscles that carry digested food through your intestines and the ring of muscles in your lower esophagus that ordinarily hold food and acids down in your stomach are both relaxed by this hormone. Try eating smaller meals more often throughout the day, and stay away from fatty, spicy, and acidic foods to ease heartburn (such as citrus fruits). Increase your fiber intake and hydration intake to help with constipation and keep things flowing more easily. Moving things forward will also need physical exertion.

Haemorrhoids. Known as varicose veins, haemorrhoids are enlarged blue or purple veins that develop around the anus. Because more blood is flowing through them and there is more pressure from the expanding uterus, these veins may swell during pregnancy. Varicose veins may irritate and cause discomfort. Try relaxing in a warm tub or sitz bath to ease them. When using an over-the-counter hemorrhoid ointment, check with your doctor first.

Leg pains. During the second trimester, you could experience cramping and contractions in your leg muscles. This often occurs at night. It's not apparent why they occur. Stretching your legs before night, exercising often, consuming foods high in magnesium, such as beans or whole grains, drinking plenty of water, consuming the proper calcium intake, and wearing comfortable shoes are all ways to avoid cramps. Stretching, cold, heat, or massage may assist to relieve leg cramps.

Quickening. If you aren't feeling your baby move yet, don't panic. By the halfway point of your pregnancy (20 weeks), you will likely have begun to feel the first small flutters of movement in your belly, which is often termed "quickening." Some pregnant ladies don't start to accelerate until the sixth month.

Skin alterations. Due to fluctuating hormone levels, pregnant women often seem to be "glowing" because their facial skin has a flushed appearance. Brown markings on the face, often known as the "mask of pregnancy," and a dark line (the linea nigra) running down the center of the belly may also result from an increase in the melanin pigment. After the baby is delivered, all of these skin alterations should disappear. You may cover them up with cosmetics in the meanwhile.

Wear a broad-spectrum (UVA/UVB protection) sunscreen with an SPF of at least 50 anytime you go outdoors since your skin is now more susceptible to the sun. Spend as little time in the sun as possible, especially before 10 a.m. between noon and two o'clock, dressed in long-sleeved clothing, pants, a wide-brimmed hat, and sunglasses. Additionally, you might see thin, reddish-purple lines on your thighs, breasts, or abdomen. As your skin stretches to make room for your expanding belly, stretch marks appear. There is little proof that the numerous creams and lotions that claim to prevent or get rid of stretch marks do so. Your skin might become softer and feel less itchy by using a moisturizer. After you give birth, most stretch marks should go away on their own.

Varicose and spider veins. Your blood flow has improved so that more blood can be delivered to your developing baby. Small red veins known as spider veins may develop on your skin as a result of the excessive blood flow. Once your kid is delivered, these veins should ultimately disappear. Your developing baby's pressure on your legs may also reduce blood flow to your lower body, resulting in bulging, blue, or purple veins in your legs. They are referred to as varicose veins. While there is no way to eliminate varicose veins, you can stop them from growing worse by being active throughout the day and elevating your legs on a stool if you must remain still for extended periods. For more support, put on a support hose. After giving birth, varicose veins should start to get better after three months.

Infection in the urinary tract. The second trimester is a typical time for bacterial infections of the bladder or urinary system, which are located above the uterus. They are brought on by alterations to your urinary system or a developing uterus that makes it more difficult to empty your bladder.

You might have symptoms like lower abdominal ache, pain or burning when you urinate, frequent urges to urinate, hazy or odorous urine, pain during sex, or traces of blood or mucus in your urine. See your doctor as soon as possible since bladder infections may spread to your kidneys and lead to early delivery or low-weight kids. To identify the illness and treat it, they will give you a urine analysis and a urine culture.

Weight increase. By the end of the first trimester, morning sickness often subsides. Your appetite should recover and perhaps increase after that. Be mindful of how much you're eating even when the meal seems much more enticing. During the second trimester, you just need an additional 300 to 500 calories per day, and you should grow between half and one pound each week.

Emergencies Signs

Any of these signs and symptoms might indicate a problem with your pregnancy. Don't wait until your prenatal appointment to bring it up. If you have call your doctor immediately away.

Jaundice, severe dizziness, vomiting, or severe abdominal cramps.

Too little weight growth or rapid weight increase (greater than 6.5 pounds per month) (less than 10 pounds at 20 weeks into the pregnancy)

a lot of perspiration

During the second trimester, the baby growth

Your baby may gain up to 3 pounds of weight and up to 16 inches in length during the second trimester. Their brain and other organs expand and mature considerably.

A day, their heart pumps 100 quarts of blood. Despite having completely developed lungs, they are not yet ready to breathe. Additionally, your unborn child can move, turn, swallow, and hear your voice while still inside of you.

The eyes and ears on your baby's head shift into the proper locations. Their eyelids have a range of motion. The infant has a regular sleep and waking cycle. They develop eyebrows and eyelashes.

Nails on the baby's fingers and toes develop. Little toes and fingers separate. Their toeprints and fingerprints become distinctive.

Your baby's head develops hair. They also develop lanugo, or downy, fine hair, all over their bodies. The vernix caseosa is a protective layer that covers their body and is creamy, white, and finally absorbed by their skin. By this period, the placenta in your unborn child has finished developing. The placenta is an organ that provides oxygen and nutrition to the fetus. It also gets rid of the trash. Additionally, during the second trimester, your foetus starts to put on body fat.

In your second trimester nutrition guide

Healthy eating habits throughout pregnancy are essential for the mother and unborn child. The fetus will get the nutrients it needs to grow normally if it consumes a healthy diet.

Preventing pregnancy issues including preterm delivery, high blood pressure, and preeclampsia is another benefit of healthy eating.

Women should make sure they consume enough vitamins, minerals, proteins, fats, and carbs throughout pregnancy to promote good development. However, during the second trimester, the body requires a few more calories.

You should keep up a healthy diet throughout the second trimester. The most crucial nutrients for a pregnant person are the following:

Iron. Iron aids in the movement of oxygen inside the body. Iron serves as the baby's oxygen source throughout pregnancy.

Anemia, which raises the risk of issues including preterm delivery and postpartum depression, may be brought on by a diet low in iron.

When pregnant, 27 milligrams of iron per day are advised (mg).

Several sources of iron are:
Fatty meat, prepared seafood, green leafy veggies, nuts, lentils and beans, entire grains, such as oatmeal and bread

Iron from animal sources is absorbed by the body more effectively than iron from plant-based sources.

So, those who don't consume meat may increase absorption rates by consuming vitamin C-rich meals at the same time.

Oranges, orange juice, strawberries, and tomatoes are all sources of vitamin C.

Try to avoid consuming calcium-rich meals or supplements at the same time as foods containing iron. Iron absorption is decreased by calcium.

Protein. To support the baby's brain and other tissue growth in the latter stages of pregnancy, women should try to consume 1.52 grams (g) per kilogram (kg) of body weight each day. A lady who weighs 79 kg (175 pounds), for instance, should strive to consume 121 g of protein per day.

Protein is also required for the mother's uterus and breasts to develop.

Among the best sources of protein are:

Eggs, cooked, not raw, fish, peas, beans, and lentils, as well as lean meats, almonds, tofu, and tempeh

Calcium. 1,000 mg of calcium per day is the recommended dietary intake during pregnancy. Pregnant people under the age of 18 should try to have 1,300 mg of calcium per day.

The development of the baby's bones and teeth is aided by calcium, which also contributes to the health of the baby's muscles, nerves, and circulatory system.

Foods high in calcium include:

White beans, almonds, sardines, salmon, dairy (milk, yogurt, and pasteurized cheese), eggs, and (with bones)

Greens like broccoli, kale, and turnip greens

Folat. Dark green leafy vegetables, whole grains, and oranges all contain folate.

B vitamin folate is. Folic acid is the name for folate's synthetic version.

Due to its ability to lower the risk of preterm labor and prevent neural tube disorders such as spina bifida, folate is crucial throughout pregnancy.

The incidence of congenital cardiac abnormalities is greatly reduced by folic acid, according to a review of 18 research. But additional study is still required.

Women should have 400 to 800 micrograms (mcg) of folic acid or folate per day while they are pregnant and before. The most reliable sources are:

Other legumes with black-eyed peas

enriched grains

Dark green leafy vegetables, such as collard Greens, spinach, and cabbage

Oranges

Whole grains, like rice

Prenatal vitamins or folic acid supplements should be used before and throughout pregnancy since there is no assurance that a person would get enough folate from dietary sources to satisfy their daily needs.

A baby's growing bones and teeth are strengthened by vitamin D. A daily dosage of 600 International Units (IU) is advised during pregnancy.

 Many individuals may fulfill part of their vitamin D requirements since the body can produce it from sunlight. However, estimates indicate that owing to lack of sun exposure and other causes, more than 40% of the adult population in the United States may be vitamin D deficient.

Few naturally occurring foods contain vitamin D, but fortified foods like milk and cereal do.

Foods that are rich in vitamin D include:

Salmon, fresh tuna, and mackerel are examples of fatty fish,

Beef liver, cheese, egg yolks, fish liver oils,

Sun-exposed mushrooms,

Enhanced juices and other beverages.

Additionally offered are vitamin D pills, which are beneficial for those who do not reside in an area with abundant sunshine.

Fatty acids omega-3. Omega-3 fats in the diet provide advantages for both the mother and the child. The heart, brain, eyes, immune system, and central nervous system are supported by these vital fatty acids. Omega-3 may delay preterm labor, reduce the chance of preeclampsia, and lessen the possibility of postpartum depression.

During pregnancy, 1.4 g of omega-3 fats per day is the recommended amount. Contains omega-3 fatty acids include:

Salmon, mackerel, fresh tuna, herring, sardines, and other oily fish,

Fatty fish,

Flaxseeds,

the chia seed.

Omega-3 in seeds comes in a form that the body must change to use it. Each person's body is capable of doing this to a different degree.

Vegans and vegetarians who want to acquire the omega-3s they need while pregnant may need to take a supplement made of algae.

Water. To keep hydrated, pregnant persons need more water than non-pregnant people do. The amniotic sac and placenta are formed with the aid of water. Pregnancy issues including neural tube abnormalities and decreased breast milk production may be exacerbated by dehydration.

To avoid dehydration and associated problems, pregnant women should drink at least 8 to 12 glasses of water each day.

Noxious foods

Soft cheeses must be avoided when pregnant.

The following foods should be avoided by a person when pregnant:

Raw fish, raw eggs, and raw meat,

High mercury-content fish, such as swordfish, shark, tilefish, and king mackerel,

Dairy products without pasteurization, Brie, blue cheese, and feta are examples of soft cheeses.

Since there is no established safe threshold for alcohol consumption during pregnancy, it should be avoided. Alcohol may be detrimental in all forms and may result in:

miscarriage and stillbirth.

Fetal alcohol spectrum disorders (FASDs) are illnesses that result in mental, behavioral, and physical impairments.

Caffeine may be used by pregnant women in moderation. Although the American Pregnancy Association advises pregnant women to avoid caffeine as much as possible, experts say it is okay to ingest 150 to 300 mg daily.

Between 95 to 165 mg of caffeine are present in an 8-ounce cup of coffee, while around 45 mg are present in a 6-ounce drink of black tea. Caffeine may also be found in cola drinks, chocolate, green tea, and certain medicines.

How Much Should You Eat?

Gaining weight during pregnancy is completely normal and healthy. The body's increased blood volume, the presence of amniotic fluid, and the weight of the baby all contribute to an individual's weight gain.

During the second and third trimesters, the body needs 300 more calories per day to control this weight increase.

In the second trimester, women who started their pregnancies at a healthy weight normally gain 1 to 2 pounds each week. The risk of issues, such as high blood pressure, a bigger baby, and cesarean birth, rises when a person gains more weight than is healthy.

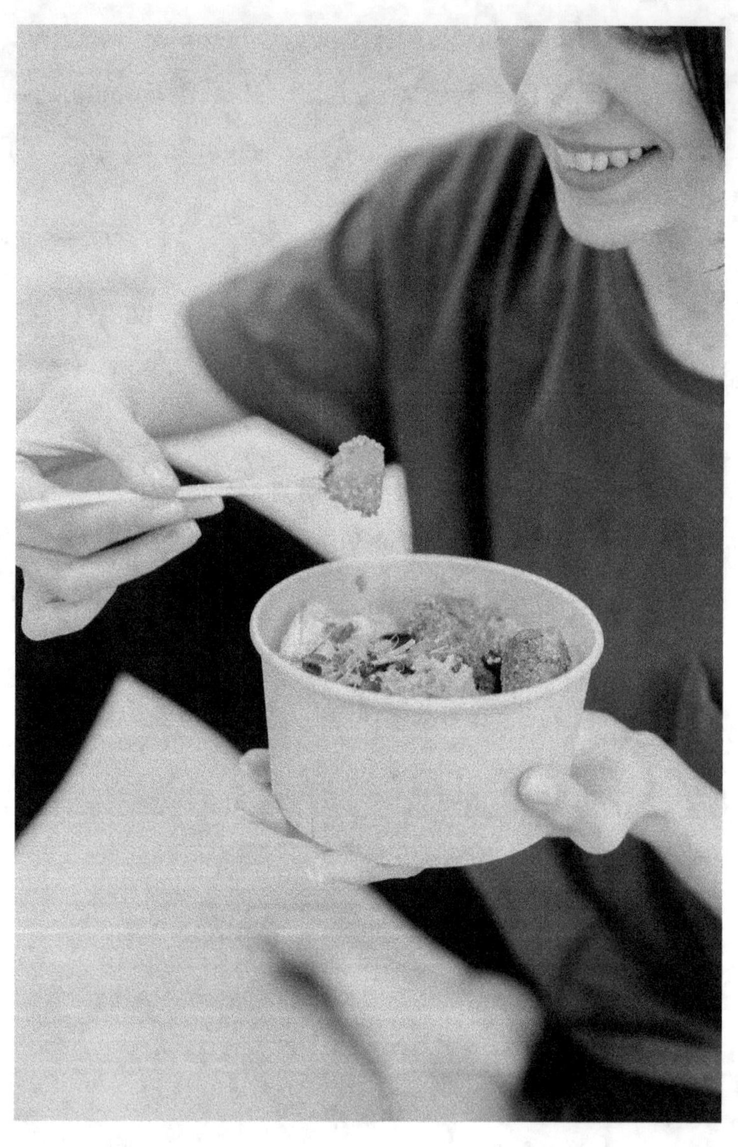

Chapter 4: What to do and what to expect during the third trimester.

An average pregnancy lasts for 40 weeks. Three trimesters are formed from the weeks. The third trimester of pregnancy lasts from weeks 28 to 40.

For a pregnant woman, the third trimester may be emotionally and physically taxing. After week 37, the baby is regarded as full term, and delivery is only a matter of time. You may lessen any worry you may have during the last few weeks of your pregnancy by doing some research and learning what to anticipate throughout the third trimester.

Changes that come along with third trimester

A woman may feel additional aches, pains, and swelling in the third trimester as she carries the baby inside of her. Additionally, a pregnant woman may start feeling nervous about giving birth.

A lot of baby movement, infrequent, absolutely random tightening of the uterus (called Braxton-Hicks contractions), which are typically not painful, more frequent trips to the toilet, heartburn, swollen ankles, fingers, or face, and hemorrhoids.
watery milk that might flow from delicate breasts and trouble sleeping

If you experience any of the following, call your doctor right away. Excruciating contractions that are becoming more frequent and intensely painful bleeding whenever you feel like it excessive edema fast weight gain
What occurs to the developing fetus in the third trimester?

Your baby's bones are completely developed at week 32. Now that its eyes are open, the infant can also see light. The body of the newborn will start to retain minerals like calcium and iron.

The infant should be lying head down by week 36. Your doctor may suggest a cesarean delivery if the baby doesn't shift into this position or may attempt to alter the baby's position. To deliver the baby, the doctor makes an incision in the mother's abdomen and uterus at this point.

Your baby is full term and its organs are prepared to operate independently after week 37. The baby is now between 19 and 21 inches long, and the Office on Women's HealthTrusted Source estimates that it weighs between 6 and 9 pounds.

From the doctor

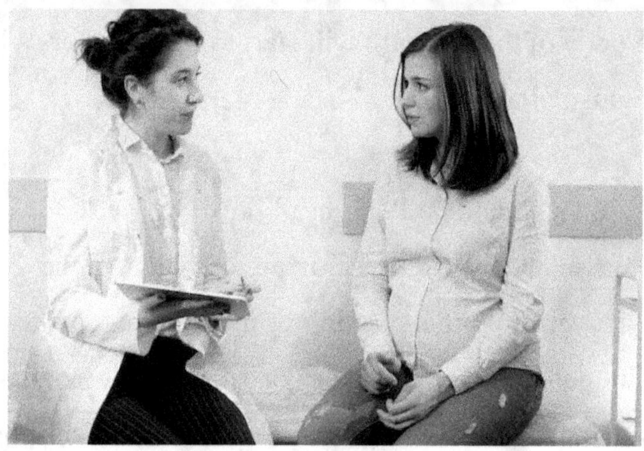

During the third trimester, you will see your doctor more often. Your doctor could do a Group B strep test around week 36 to check for a bacteria that can be highly dangerous to an unborn child. If your test is positive, your doctor will prescribe antibiotics.

A vaginal exam will be used by your doctor to monitor your development. As your due date approaches, your cervix will thin and soften to aid in the opening of the delivery canal.

How to to maintain your health in the third trimester

As your pregnancy progresses, it's critical to know what to do and what to avoid to look after both you and your growing child.

Maintain your prenatal vitamin intake. Unless you are in discomfort or have edema, keep moving.

By doing Kegel exercises, you may strengthen your pelvic floor.

Consume a diet rich in fiber, low-fat protein sources, fruits, and vegetables.

Get plenty of water.

Consume enough energy (about 300 more calories than normal per day).

Keep moving by walking.

Maintain good oral and gum health. Premature labor has been related to poor tooth hygiene.

Rest and sleep as much as you can.

Things to avert

Engaging in vigorous exercise or weight training that might harm your stomach, alcohol, or caffeine (no more than one cup of coffee or tea per day)

using illicit drugs

smoked fish or raw seafood

White snapper fish, sharks, swordfish, or mackerel (they have high levels of mercury)

raw sprouts unpasteurized milk or other dairy products, which may contain a parasite that causes toxoplasmosis

hot dogs or deli meats

following prescription medicines: Long vehicle rides and flights, if at all feasible, with isotretinoin (Accutane) for acne, acitretin (Soriatane) for psoriasis, thalidomide (Thalomid), and ACE inhibitors for high blood pressure (after 34 weeks, airlines may not let you board the plane because of the possibility of an unexpected delivery on the plane)

If you must travel, get some exercise by taking a short stroll every hour or two.

Getting ready

Choose the location of your baby's birth if you haven't previously. These last-minute measures may facilitate a smoother delivery.

If you haven't already, take a prenatal class. This is a chance to learn about the various delivery methods and what to anticipate during labor.

Find a friend or family member who can look after your other kids or pets.

Prepare some foods that you can freeze and consume when the baby comes home.

Prepare an overnight bag with supplies for both you and your infant.

When traveling to the hospital, plan your route and form of transportation.

Create a birth plan: Together with your doctor, create a birth plan. This might include making decisions about who you want to assist you in the delivery room, any worries you have about hospital protocols and pre-registering with your insurance details.

Make maternity leave arrangements with your company.
Prepare a crib for your infant and make sure it is secure and up to date.
Make that any "hand-me-down" items, such as cribs and strollers, adhere to current government safety regulations. Get a fresh car seat.

Verify the functionality of the carbon monoxide and smoke detectors in your house.
Keep a list of emergency numbers, including poison control, close to hand.
Purchase plenty of diapers, wipes, and infant clothes in several sizes.

Nutrition needed

During the third trimester, your baby swiftly puts on weight and continues to develop. Things like eyes opening, the formation of nails, and the growth of hair are only a few examples.

Given all that is going on, it is crucial for your baby's health that you make the right nutritional choices.
The components of your meals and snacks need to be:
Protein, fruits, and vegetables
whole grains
wholesome oils and fats
Pasteurised dairy products with reduced or no fat
You can find the vitamins, minerals, and nutrients you need each day in those items.

Your baby's growing bones benefit from vitamin A. Both their skin and eyesight are supported by it. During the third trimester, your baby's eyes open and begin to sense light.

Vitamin A may be found in: Dairy products, fish, Sweet potatoes, spinach, cantaloupe, carrots, and fortified cereals

Your body can absorb iron better with vitamin C. Additionally, it promotes the health of your baby's bones, gums, and teeth. Your immune system also needs it.

Citrus fruits including oranges, tangerines, grapefruit, Kiwi, strawberries, tomatoes, red and green peppers, and broccoli are all good sources of vitamin C.

Red blood cells and the brain of your unborn child both benefit from vitamin B6, which is a crucial nutrient. It's in:

Red blood cell production and nervous system health are both supported by vitamin B12. Since B12 is not naturally present in plant foods, vegans and vegetarians must take a B12 supplement. Before using any supplement, consult your doctor.

Your baby and you can better absorb calcium with vitamin D. This supports the development of your baby's teeth and bones. It is available from:

Your body may more easily absorb iron from foods and supplements with vitamin C.

Iodine aids in brain development in infants. Seafood, dairy, grain goods, and iodized salt are all sources of iodine.

Folate and folic acid help shield your unborn child against problems with the brain and spinal cord known as neural tube defects. The placenta and your unborn child both depend on them for growth in your body. Beef liver, peanuts, dark green leafy vegetables, almonds, peas, beans, fortified morning cereals, enriched bread, pasta, flour, rice, cornmeal, oranges, and orange juice are among the foods you may find them in.

Your baby's brain develops with the aid of omega-3 fatty acids. They may be found in many fish. Make careful to choose seafood low in mercury, such as cod, herring, trout, and salmon.

You are allowed to have 8–12 ounces of white (albacore) tuna every week, but no more than 6 ounces should be consumed in a single week. If you consume more than that, there is a danger that your bloodstream may get too contaminated with mercury. The development of your baby's nervous system and brain may be impacted by this.

Flaxseed, walnuts, chia seeds, cantaloupe, broccoli, spinach, and kidney beans are other omega-3-rich foods. Protein aids in your baby's growth and the production of blood in both your and your baby's body. It is available from:

Lean meat, poultry, seafood, cottage cheese, egg whites, lentils, nuts, beans, seeds, and peas are all good options. Soy-based goods
Less than 30% of your calories should come from fats and oils. But they do provide significant advantages.

They provide you with energy and support the growth of the placenta and the organs of your unborn child.

Eat less fat-containing food, such as meat and whole-milk dairy products.

An excellent supply of fiber, energy, and carbohydrates is whole grains. Mom's constipation may be relieved by all of those items. You should consume whole grains, such as those found in brown rice, oats, quinoa, barley, bulgur, whole-wheat pasta, whole-grain bread, and cereal, for at least half of your daily calorie intake.

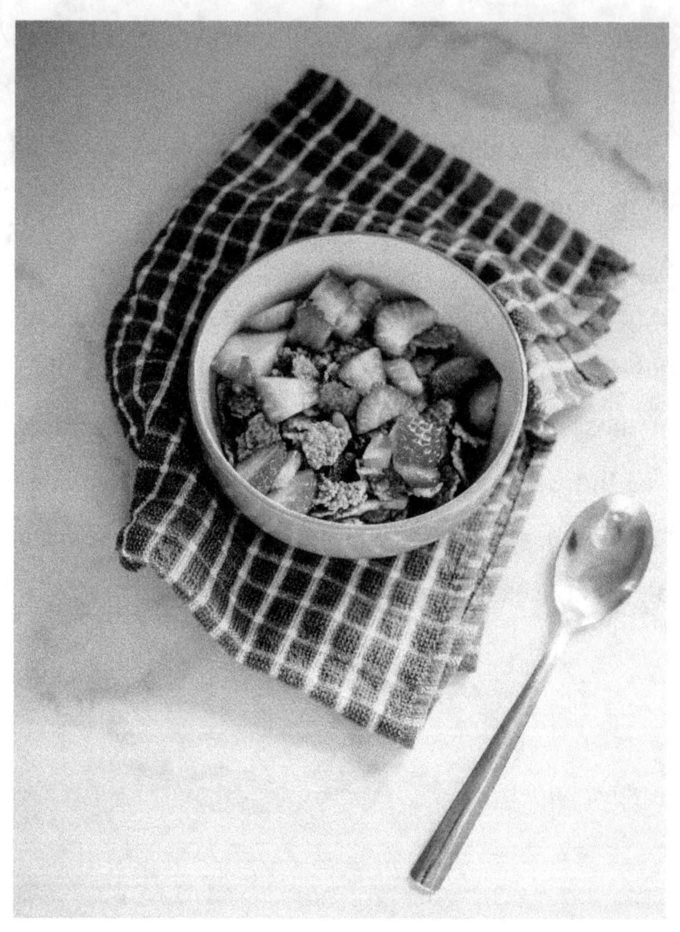

fortified cereals

Chapter 5: Comfortable sleeping position for pregnant mom

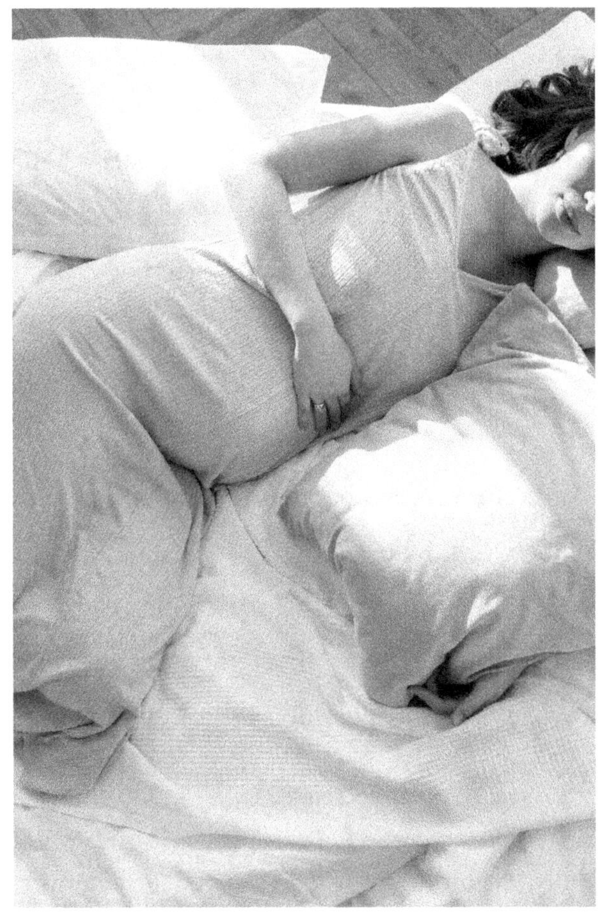

Many women question how to sleep comfortably while expecting. Having trouble sleeping is normal during pregnancy, particularly in the third trimester when it may be difficult to find a comfortable posture. Some expectant women may also fear that certain body postures could harm the unborn child or themselves.

Pregnant ladies who want to sleep better should use certain techniques. We explore sleep aids that are safe to use while pregnant and look at sleeping postures to attempt or avoid.

Ideal postures for sleeping

Back discomfort may be relieved by sleeping with a cushion between the legs.

It is okay for a woman to sleep on her back, side, or stomach throughout the first trimester in whichever position she finds most comfortable. Any arrangement of the aforementioned roles is acceptable.

Sleep disruption is not caused by the uterus's size. However, hormonal changes, hunger at night, nausea, and other pregnancy symptoms might make it more challenging to fall asleep.

It is recommended for women to sleep on their left side when they enter their second and third trimesters. This posture increases blood flow to the uterus while sparing the liver from pressure. Pregnant women who have hip or back discomfort may discover that putting one or two pillows between their knees or bending their knees as they sleep will help them feel better.

A lady may switch to this posture if she wants to sleep on her right side. There is no evidence to support the notion that something is risky.

Other sleeping positions that might assist with common problems include:
To lessen heartburn, raise the upper body with a couple of cushions.
utilizing a body pillow or pregnant pillow to cradle the body and offer extra back support elevating the legs using cushions to relieve leg discomfort and edema

Sleeping aids

When navigating the journey of pregnancy, the quest for restful sleep can become a priority. Pregnancy pillows, shaped to support the curves of the body, can alleviate discomfort and promote better sleep by providing additional support to the abdomen, back, and hips. Experiment with different pillow

For expecting mothers, ensuring a good night's sleep is crucial for overall well-being. While it's essential to prioritize natural sleep practices, some pregnant women may face challenges in finding a comfortable sleeping position. To enhance sleep quality, consider using pregnancy pillows designed to provide support for the changing contours of the body. Additionally, practicing relaxation techniques and establishing a consistent sleep routine can contribute to more restful nights. Always consult with your healthcare provider before using any sleep aids to ensure they are safe during pregnancy.

Furthermore, establishing a calming bedtime routine can signal to your body that it's time to wind down. This may include activities such as gentle stretching, reading, or listening to soothing music. Avoiding stimulants like caffeine in the evening and creating a comfortable sleep environment can also contribute to a more tranquil night.

Investing in a new mattress is one of the greatest ways to follow the experts' recommendations for how many hours a pregnant woman should sleep. You can relax at night, fall asleep more quickly, and remain asleep longer with the aid of a comfortable, supportive mattress.
Being as constant as you can with your sleep routine is a certain approach to determine for yourself how many hours of sleep you need, we know this may be difficult.

If sleep troubles persist, it's advisable to consult your healthcare provider. They can offer personalized guidance and ensure that any interventions, such as over-the-counter sleep aids, are safe for use during pregnancy. Remember, prioritizing rest is a key element in nurturing both your well-being and that of your growing baby.

During Trimester Sleep

First Trimester

Your body goes through a lot of changes throughout the first trimester, both psychologically and physically.

Your body is still under a lot of stress, even if you are less active throughout the day. Without making up for this tension, you'll rapidly tire yourself.

In the same way that first-time moms should organize their day, they should also plan their sleep.

If you think you might use a sleep, schedule one. Additionally, go to bed every night at the same time, even if you don't immediately fall asleep, to help your body adjust to the new schedule.

Second Trimester

Your sleep may become better during the second trimester of your pregnancy than it did during the first.

You could feel more energized now that your body has adjusted to the alterations that began in the first three months. Don't allow this fresh energy to interfere with your regular sleep patterns!

Don't give in to the urge to fill your day with activities simply because you feel better. And by all means, keep getting as much rest as you can.

Thrid Trimester

When it comes to the issue of how many hours a pregnant woman should sleep each night, the third trimester is the hardest of the three.

The last three months have been filled with issues that will prevent you from obtaining the eight to ten hours of sleep you need to feel your best, including back discomfort, difficulties getting comfortable, and your baby kicking at unusual hours.

If your schedule allows, take a nap if you discover that you are becoming drowsy in the middle of the day due to inadequate sleep the previous night.

Additionally, as we have indicated, try not to worry about how much sleep you're getting at this time. You already have enough to worry about! Simply try to get as much sleep as you can.

Limit daytime naps.
As we previously indicated, taking sleep throughout the day may become a necessary component of your daily routine. I understand. Just keep your naps brief to avoid having trouble going to sleep at night.
The majority of people find that midday is the optimum time for naps, but determine the schedule that works best for you. Set a timer for 20 to 40 minutes, but don't let it go above an hour, and then get some rest.

To avoid being too stimulated at night to have trouble falling asleep, think about completing a small workout after you wake up.

How to Avoid Nausea Before Bed

During pregnancy, morning sickness may strike at any moment. Your sleep schedule is severely harmed when it happens at night.

Try eating some crackers a few minutes before you lay down to minimize nausea before night.
A few crackers should be kept close to your bed in case you wake up sick in the middle of the night.

Cut down on late-night bathroom breaks
When your child is old enough, they will sometimes press on your bladder. You could discover that you need to get up many times throughout the night to use the bathroom!

Even while you can't stop your child from using your bladder as a punching bag, you can cut down on the quantity of liquid you consume in the evenings to reduce the number of overnight toilet visits.

Drink lots of water during the day, but three to four hours before going to bed, stop. As a result, your bladder won't be as full in the middle of the night. This will allow your body time to process a significant amount of the water out of your system.

For the emotional and physical well-being of your family, taking care of yourself and your infant is essential.

Chapter 6: How to ensure a safe delivery

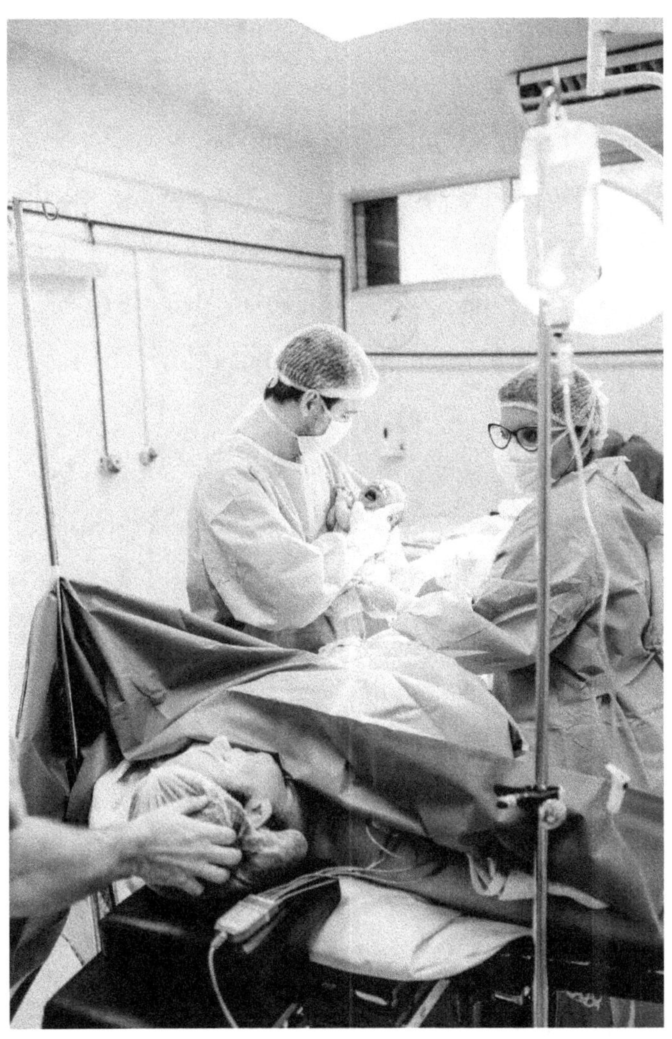

The natural method of giving birth, normal delivery is often safer for both the mother and the child. However, some ladies choose to have a c-section because they worry about the discomfort of labor.

According to research, 85% of pregnant women may give birth naturally, and just 15% may need a c-section for medical reasons. However, data indicate that more than 30% of pregnant women have an elective cesarean birth, indicating that this procedure has grown common.

A c-section may seem like the simpler option, but it comes with a lengthy recovery time and the potential for difficulties both before and after delivery. Therefore, a good distribution method should only be selected after weighing the benefits and drawbacks.

What Is the Natural Delivery?

Natural delivery is a healthy technique to bring the child into the world. Unless you have certain medical issues, giving birth naturally and normally is not difficult. The natural birthing process also contributes to a healthy baby and a quick recovery for the new mother.

Although there is no magic trick or a quick way to birth normally, there are several things you may do to increase your chances.

Elements That Increase Your Possibility Of A Natural Delivery.

Your capacity to experience a routine delivery depends on several circumstances. However, they may not promise a success rate of 100%. Your chances of having a normal delivery may be higher if:

In your prior pregnancies, if you had a typical vaginal birth.

You don't suffer from any underlying medical conditions that can become worse during pregnancy or childbirth, such as asthma.

You are the right weight since being overweight might raise the likelihood of having a big baby and decrease the likelihood of having a healthy pregnancy.

regular delivery.

Your pregnancy is progressing without any problems.

Throughout your pregnancy, you are physically active. The likelihood of a normal birth increases with physical fitness.

You have power over your physiological circumstances, such as blood pressure, blood sugar, and hemoglobin.

The prenatal general health issues listed above affect your likelihood of having a normal delivery. You might also follow some advice that can improve your chances of having a normal delivery.

Advice For Natural Delivery

The ideal delivery method for both mother and child is normal vaginal birth. And if you want to go natural, you might use this advice (4) for a better result:

Avoid becoming stressed: Stress is a typical side effect of pregnancy. Avoiding worry, anxiety, and uncontrollable thinking is recommended since these emotions may make labor a nightmarish experience.

Try any meditation technique that makes you feel at ease.

Do visualization exercises, read books, and listen to music.

Keep association with kind and decent individuals.

Avoid those who or things that give you a bad or unpleasant feeling.

Avoid unpleasant birth stories and maintain your good attitude: There might be both straightforward and challenging delivery stories, You can get a panic attack if you continue to listen to unfavorable reports.

Simply walk away from a mother if she happens to be sharing her unpleasant birthing story.

Tell rumor-mongers no.

Keep in mind that not everyone's experience with labor is the same. It does not necessarily follow that you will have a difficult delivery because your buddy did.

Become knowledgeable about giving birth:

The power of knowledge is vast. Learn everything you can about labor and delivery procedures.

Consult your doctor to have all of your questions regarding pregnancy and delivery answered.

Read birth-related literature.

Speak to your mother and other experienced women in the family who can aid you.

Learn about natural stress-reduction methods including breathing exercises and coping mechanisms.

Create a solid network of allies: possess enough emotional support. Bring your spouse, mother, and close friends so they can encourage you and ease your worries about a routine birth.

When it comes to labor, be sure you and your spouse are on the same page.

Your family will support you, but if you have any opposing opinions or beliefs on pregnancy, be sure to discuss them with them and reach an understanding.

A strong support network may help reduce stress.

Pick your doctor carefully: It is a sad reality that many physicians pressure moms to undergo a C-section out of convenience. Therefore, it's crucial to choose a doctor who will properly handle your pregnancy.

Make sure the clinic and your doctor have a high rate of typical deliveries.Ask your doctor what he or she thinks about a typical birth.

Find a new doctor if you believe your current one may not respect your desire for a regular birth.

Hire a doula with experience: Finding a skilled doula to assist you with birthing is half the fight won!

Having a skilled doula at your side may be helpful.

She can support you throughout childbirth and keep you calm.

She assists you in nursing the newborn after the delivery.

Remain hydrated: Now that you are pregnant, water is even more important for your health.

Your body will work hard throughout labor, so drink more water to keep hydrated. Water gives your body a lot of energy and stamina, so you won't likely require IV fluids.

To meet your daily need for fluids, you may also stock up on some fresh juices or healthy energy drinks. One of the finest pieces of advice for a typical delivery is this.

Hydrotherapy: You may utilize water for more than just drinking; you can also use it to speed up work. Hydrotherapy helps ease labor-related discomfort and agony while also assisting in reducing stress.

To relieve tension, fill the bathtub with water and soak. Showers, birthing pools, and hot compresses may all be used to reduce discomfort and promote relaxation.

To protect your unborn child from any injury, keep the water at room temperature.

The ice game: Try the ice game that includes your spouse if you want to learn the best ways to handle the birthing process.

Everybody takes a turn holding an ice cube for 60 seconds.

Try chatting to each other while holding the ice cube the first time.

Try walking around while holding the ice cube next.

Hold an ice cube for 60 seconds while being completely silent.

It is an excellent approach to determine how long you can tolerate and handle labor discomfort.

Pay attention to your postures: So that the baby may slide easily, keep your body in alignment. Your body may go out of alignment if you stand or sit for long periods, sleep in an uncomfortable posture, or wear tight-fitting clothing and high heels.

Sit with your back properly supported. Your spine would be under more strain during pregnancy, and mistreating your body would make the discomfort worse.

Sit with your legs folded or spread out since dangling your legs too long might cause edema.

When sitting or bending to lift anything, avoid slouching. Avoid rushing up or down the steps.

Try to avoid gaining too much weight: Yes, it's crucial to gain a healthy amount of weight when you're pregnant, but you don't have to pack on the pounds. Women who are overweight may have difficulties giving birth and need a C-section.

Obesity might make it difficult to keep an eye on the baby throughout labor, complicating a routine delivery.
If you are fat, your baby may be large and difficult to deliver

Visit a chiropractor for adjustments: Some individuals support chiropractic adjustments, while others oppose them. But if you try it and have excellent results with frequent chiropractic appointments, you can keep doing it.

Stress relief via chiropractic adjustments is possible.

A skilled practitioner may relieve pinched nerves as well as stiff, aching muscles.

With frequent adjustments, you may also reduce back discomfort and strengthen your thighs and back. It may be quite beneficial with a routine birth.

An unaligned pelvis may be corrected with chiropractic adjustments, which can aid with normal birth.

In the first and second trimesters, you may see a chiropractor once per month, and more often in the third trimester.

Food Advice For Easy Delivery

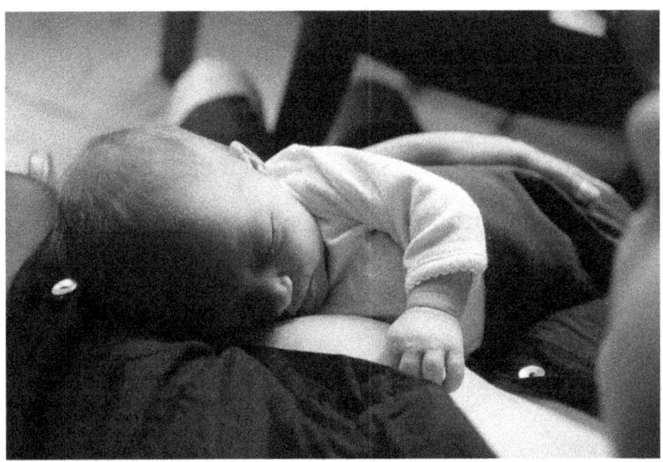

Your nutrition is crucial for maintaining your health and allowing for a natural delivery.

Eat sensibly: A healthy mother will produce a healthy child.

A balanced diet should include plenty of fruits, vegetables, lean meat, legumes, and dairy products.

Pick foods that are high in protein, starchy meals in moderation, and dark green veggies.

Make sure you consume an iron-rich diet since your body requires more iron when you are pregnant.

Don't consume organic meat.

Eat nothing that contains retinol.

Moderate seafood consumption is advised.

Reduce your sugar consumption.

Steer clear of consuming street food since it may include germs that are harmful to your health.

Include foods high in bromelain: An enzyme called bromelain can induce labor and soften the cervix.

Fruits with high bromelain content include mango and pineapple.

For optimal benefits, eat raw bromelain-rich foods.

However, avoid eating too many of these fruits since you can go into labor too soon.

Consume spicy food: Although it may be an old wives' tale, many ladies believe in this tactic.

Spicy meals might increase body temperature and promote proper delivery.

However, eating spicy food might cause severe indigestion, heartburn, and diarrhea in certain women. Avoid this and try something else if it applies to you!

Exercise is always beneficial for everyone. Being physically active throughout pregnancy promotes a natural birth.

Exercises During Pregnancy For A Normal Delivery

Never start an exercise program without consulting your doctor beforehand. The greatest person to advise you on which workouts could benefit your body is your doctor. Here are some common delivery exercises that can both strengthen your pelvic floor and assist your baby in achieving the ideal birthing position.

Practice appropriate breathing techniques: You hardly even pay attention to your breathing. However, it is the only item that has the potential to simplify labor altogether and eliminate the need for a C-section.

The following breathing techniques are for normal delivery:
inhaling via the chest
Taking a breath from the stomach
sluggish breathing
Breathing deeply and shallowly in turn

Swimming and walking: Both forms of exercise are highly advised for expectant mothers.
A great low-intensity workout is walking. So put on a pair of comfortable sneakers and start moving. You may

spend at least 30 minutes each day walking around your home or in your garden. Constipation, high blood pressure, and restlessness issues are all prevented by it.

Another fantastic exercise you can do to prepare for a typical delivery is swimming. It guards against muscular damage, controls heartbeat, builds muscle, and maintains your body in shape..

Routine exercise: Mild exercise will increase your stamina and keep you active throughout your pregnancy. Here are some workouts you might try:

Kegel exercises strengthen the thigh muscles and aid in reducing tension during birth.
Performing pelvic tilts and cat-and-cow stretches to relax the pelvic muscles and release the lower back.
The lower back is stretched and the pelvis is opened in the butterfly stance.
Squatting aids in opening the pelvis and positioning your baby for optimal delivery.

Pregnancy yoga: Yoga is a fantastic approach to not only have a healthy body but also to make labor easier.

The primary focus of yoga is proper breathing, which may be particularly beneficial during labor and delivery.

Pregnancy-friendly yoga positions include those that ease lower back stress.

Your hips, shoulders, and chest will expand up as a result of these stances.

To make prenatal yoga safe for you and your unborn child, enroll in lessons from a professional.

As your due date draws near, your body could indicate that it is prepared for a natural birth if these suggestions increase the likelihood of vaginal delivery.

Why Choose the Normal Delivery Method?

childbirth is a natural process for which the human body was created. Healthy women may not even need an epidural or painkillers during a C-section. Unfortunately, some medical professionals can advocate a C-section to save the suffering of laboring women rather than assuming that they would require painkillers.

Healthier for the mother and the child: The healing period is shortened with vaginal delivery. Babies immune systems are strengthened by the protective microorganisms they get via the birth canal. Expulsion of extra amniotic fluid from the lungs after delivery may also reduce the incidence of respiratory illnesses. You won't have adequate healing time if you have a cesarean birth since the subsequent contractions and uterine stimulants (such as Pitocin infusion) would be so quick and intense. The fetus receives less oxygen as a result. Additionally, epidurals may make a fever more likely, necessitating the need for antibiotics.

Helps with breastfeeding: Delivered babies effortlessly adjust to nursing. Painkillers used during C-section births are transferred to the infant via nursing. So soon after birth, the infant displays unusual sucking behavior. The infant also struggles to latch and may have an uncoordinated suck/swallow reflex for a few hours or days.

A stronger connection with the body: Without medicines, you will be attentive and aware of the approaching labor. Your body and you will be intertwined. Painkillers often make a woman feel less physically connected to the childbirth process.

Quicker recovery after birth: A quick recovery time usually follows a natural birth since no anesthetics, needles, or tubes are placed on any body parts. You can move about and exercise without it harming your health. The body creates endorphins, which are relaxing and pain-relieving substances, during normal delivery. However, the body will not create as many endorphins if painkillers are used.

Gives you a sense of assurance: Women who give birth naturally report feeling more powerful and confident. You could feel more resilient and less afraid to take on other problems that life presents.

Brief hospitalization: Although labor might be uncomfortable and draining, once it is over, it is over. One of the biggest advantages of vaginal delivery is that it requires less recovery time and hospitalization than a C-section.

Minimal surgery: Major surgery includes a C-section. Therefore, if you can give birth vaginally, you'll avoid having surgery as well as the various health hazards it entails, such as painful anesthetic responses, scars, infections, and heavy bleeding.

Quicker fusion: Exposure of skin to skin is a wonderful approach to developing a relationship with a baby. It is simpler for the mother to hold her baby after a normal birth and establish a rapid relationship.

Lower likelihood of lung issues: During a typical delivery, the muscles pushing the baby out might also force fluid from the infant's lungs. Because of this, infants delivered normally are less likely to have breathing problems.

Increasing the infant's immune system: Did you know that your baby's immune system might benefit from a routine delivery? Well, when the infant passes through the birth canal, it picks up some beneficial bacteria. The immunological and digestive systems of the infant are strengthened by this.

You may be wondering how our bodies can undergo such a complex procedure now that you are aware of the benefits of natural delivery. We will now explain it.

Symptoms And Signs Of Labor/ Delivery

A few weeks before the anticipated due date, changes might happen. Your doctor also advises you to watch out for these indicators of labor. The indications and symptoms, however, might differ from woman to woman and from pregnancy to pregnancy.

As the baby enters the pelvis, the motions become less coordinated.

Joints that are loose because the relaxin hormone softens and relaxes the pelvic area's ligaments and joints.

want to pee a lot since the baby's head is pressing on the bladder

Braxton Hicks contractions, which seem like pre-labor false contractions

Lower back cramping and discomfort when joints and muscles stretch and become active in preparation for delivery.

Your doctor will observe cervical dilation at the prenatal exam.

Watery stools when the muscles in the abdomen start to relax before birth

Early labor symptoms that start showing up days or hours before labor.

Vaginal discharge thickens and rises in volume.
Every time you pee, a portion of your mucus plug is expelled; nonetheless, the presence of thick, pinkish mucus, generally known as a "show," is a crucial indicator of the beginning of labor.

contractions that increase in intensity and frequency throughout time
lower back cramping and agony that spreads to the stomach and legs
Water bursting, also known as amniotic sac rupture
Once you notice these symptoms, be sure to keep your spouse or someone close by to keep an eye on your situation.

Advanced Labor Symptoms And Signs
A feeling of warmth in the abdomen
contractions that become worse

contractions could last for roughly 40 to 60 seconds while causing excruciating discomfort

increased back pain

Uterine bleeding

While some women enter advanced labor right away, others could experience all of the anguish that comes with a typical birth.

So why have we always placed a premium on natural birth? Discover next.

What To Expect During a Regular Delivery

Normally, there are three phases to birthing.

Stage 1: The cervix effaces and dilates throughout its three stages of latent, active, and transition.

Cervix dilates from 0 to 4 cm during the early or latent phase.

In first-time pregnancies, this first stage takes six to ten hours to complete. It may be longer or shorter in various circumstances.

The cervix thins and expands to a 3–4 cm diameter. Contractions start to happen more often, sporadically and continue for 30 to 45 seconds.

A faintly pink discharge follows abdominal pain. At this point, you could be admitted to the hospital and have your level of dilation regularly examined.

What to do

Rest and look after yourself.

Alternate periods of relaxation and exercise (for example, take a brief walk followed by a shower), consume lots of liquids and eat meals that are simple to digest.

Home is the finest place to stay (or hospital). Stop moving around so much.

Bring someone along to give you company and reassurance that you are not alone.

You may use relaxation and breathing techniques as contractions grow more intense.

For a relaxing atmosphere, ask your companion to massage your shoulders.

II. Cervical Dilation During Active Phase: 4–7 cm

In first-time pregnancies, this period may last anywhere between three and six hours, but it lasts less time in successive births.

You will experience excruciating agony and pressure in your back and abdomen with each contraction.

Now, every three to five minutes, the lower back, belly, and thighs experience contractions.

You'll have the impulse to exert extra effort and sharpen your attention. You might have brown or dark pink discharge.

What to do

Have a lot of fluids and empty your bladder.

Try to relax or practice deep breathing while taking breaks between contractions.

Frequently switching postures will keep you comfortable and help you advance.

You might request a massage from your spouse when the contractions intensify.

If your medical professional permits it, take a warm shower.

Dimming the lights and playing soft music are other ways to create a nice atmosphere.

III. Phase of Transition: Cervix Expands to 10 cm

In first-time pregnancies, this period may last 20 minutes to two hours, and it may take a shorter time in future pregnancies.

Cervical dilatation and effacement are complete.

Every three to four minutes, powerful, frequent, and painful contractions start to occur.

You'll get more lethargic, exhausted, and shivery.

There will be a strong impulse to push down because of the pressure that has built up in the vaginal and rectal areas. But hold off until your doctor gives the all-clear.

What to do

Concentrate on deep breathing and relaxation exercises.

Your practitioner will discuss strategies to help you fight the impulse to push if you have one but it is not yet the correct moment.

You should have your partner's full attention and words of encouragement.

Stage 2: The baby is delivered after being pushed out. The cervix is completely dilated when this stage starts. In first-time pregnancies, it lasts from 30 minutes to two hours, and it becomes shorter with successive deliveries. Moving from expanding to pressing, the body. The birth canal and pelvic area are traversed by the infant.

The baby's head has soft areas known as fontanels that enable the body to pass down the birth canal.

You'll experience a stinging, burning, and stretching feeling close to the vaginal entrance just before the baby comes out.

It will be simpler for you to push the baby's body out once the head has out.

The umbilical cord will be clamped and severed by your doctor.

What is helpful

Simply take a deep breath and glance to your spouse or family member for support.

Try shifting positions if the work is taking too long. You may benefit from being on all fours, side-lying, and squatting.

The strain may be felt in the perineum. The strain is relieved with warm compresses.

You'll learn the correct method to breathe and push from your practitioner. Observe their recommendations.

Stage 3: The placenta is taken out of the body.

The immediate period after the baby's delivery is known as "the afterbirth" as well. Usually, it takes between a few minutes to 30 minutes.

Your infant is cleansed, then put on the abdomen after the chord is cut.

When you experience discomfort and cramping once again, you will be urged to push out the placenta.

With your infant in your arms, you can be so overwhelmed that you fail to recognize this stage.

What to do

To give your infant skin-to-skin contact, place them on your breast. Caress, hug, and touch them.

It's time to introduce the infant to breastfeeding, which helps to constrict the uterus and lessen bleeding.

Apply a cold compress to the perineum to relieve pain and minimize swelling.

No matter how long the labor takes, the reward of holding the baby and seeing its face makes it all worthwhile. However, continue reading if you want a rough notion of how long a usual birth takes.

Possible Answers To Some Questions

1. Is it possible to determine my baby's location from his movements?

Even though an ultrasound scan is a reliable way to determine the baby's location, you may infer which side your baby is on based on motions.

Babies will kick harder toward the top of the bump while they are laying cephalic (head down). As your baby stretches its legs often later in pregnancy, you may feel like something is protruding on both sides of your bump. Babies in the breech position, when their feet are at the bottom, will kick the lowest portion of the bump.

During your weekly antenatal checks, your doctor may inform you of your baby's precise position.
You could be requested to use some natural ways to put the baby into the proper birthing position if it is in the breech position. An external cephalic version (ECV), when the obstetrician tries to turn the baby from outside the bump, may be necessary for specific circumstances.

2. How does the first hospital admission go?
You should check into a hospital as soon as it is verified that you are in labor. There would be paperwork to

complete and documents to sign, which your partner may assist you with.

Either your doctor or the midwife will do preliminary exams. There may be further procedures depending on the fetal heart rates and contraction patterns. However, the first examination includes measures of cervical dilatation, effacement, and station.

3. How are you going to know when to push?

As soon as your cervix has dilated to a ten-centimeter level, you will be urged to push. The majority of women push automatically because it makes them feel better and gives them an energy boost. Take a deep breath and hold it in your lungs, then lean forward so that your chin and knees are pointed in the direction of your chest. Your baby's delivery might take only a few minutes or many hours.

4. How agonizing is a normal delivery?

A difficult and demanding procedure, labor is. Abdominal muscles tighten as a result of the uterus contracting to force the baby out. Therefore, it applies pressure on the back, pelvic bolt, belly, perineum, vaginal area, and rectal area. All of them might cause excruciating agony and suffering that would persist until you gave birth.

In most cases, giving birth by normal delivery is safe for both mother and child. Don't worry too much about the discomfort and suffering of labor since your doctor and family will assist you to cope with the process. Instead, you may concentrate on getting ready for labor and welcoming your new child. Inform your healthcare practitioner of any worries you may have. Additionally, to improve your chances of natural delivery, strive to adhere to the advice provided above, eat healthfully, and engage in a safe activity

Chapter 7: Fruit and activities for tightening pelvic muscle

Fruits' nutritional benefits extend beyond maintaining health; certain fruits are also useful for vaginal tightness. Yes, you read it correctly; they efficiently tighten, protect, and maintain the health of your vagina.

The procedure of vaginal tightening involves contracting the pelvic muscles. The pelvic floor muscles become more flexible as a result of improving tightness.
It's crucial to remember that the amount of sex you have does not affect how stretchy your vagina is.

Several factors, including childbirth, menopause, and the unavoidable aging process, might contribute to a loose vagina. Vaginal relaxation or loosening may occur as a result of estrogen depletion.

Exercise and a balanced diet may help to strengthen the pelvic floor and restore it in the safest manner possible.

Kegel exercises: These are exercises that include contraction and relaxation of the muscles of the pelvic floor. For this exercise to be effective, your bladder must be empty. Your pelvic floor muscles should contract, then you should hold them for eight to ten counts before letting go. If you do this consistently, you'll see a significant improvement.

Leg lifts: To do this easy workout, all you need to do is lay on your back on the floor and raise your legs one at a time. Keep your legs straight and avoid bending them. Legs are raised and lowered in pairs.

Juice made from cranberries: By making urine more acidic and regulating the PH of the vaginal region, cranberries help to prevent and relieve the symptoms of urinary tract infections. They can combat the germs that cause illnesses because of their potent acidic components, which are not broken down during digestion. Fresh cranberries may be consumed by blending them with natural yogurt.

Water: For our vaginal mucous membrane to work correctly, females need to drink enough water. Drinking enough water will keep your vagina lubricated and help to reduce bad odors coming from your vagina.

Avocado: This fruit assists in re-establishing the vaginal wall and enhancing the condition of the vagina. Healthy fats found in avocados increase libido. It also contains a lot of potassium and vitamin B-6, which help to build the vaginal membrane.

Sweet potatoes: This food contains vitamin A, which supports healthy uterine and vaginal walls and aids in the production of the hormones required to maintain vigor and energy.

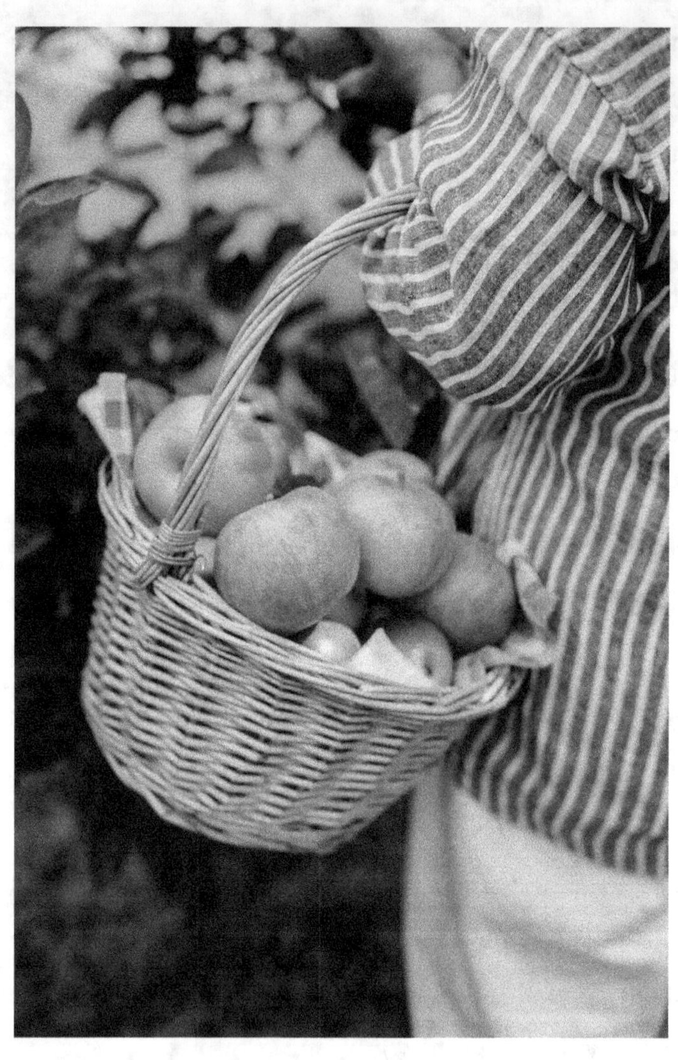

Chapter 8: Looking after your health after childbirth

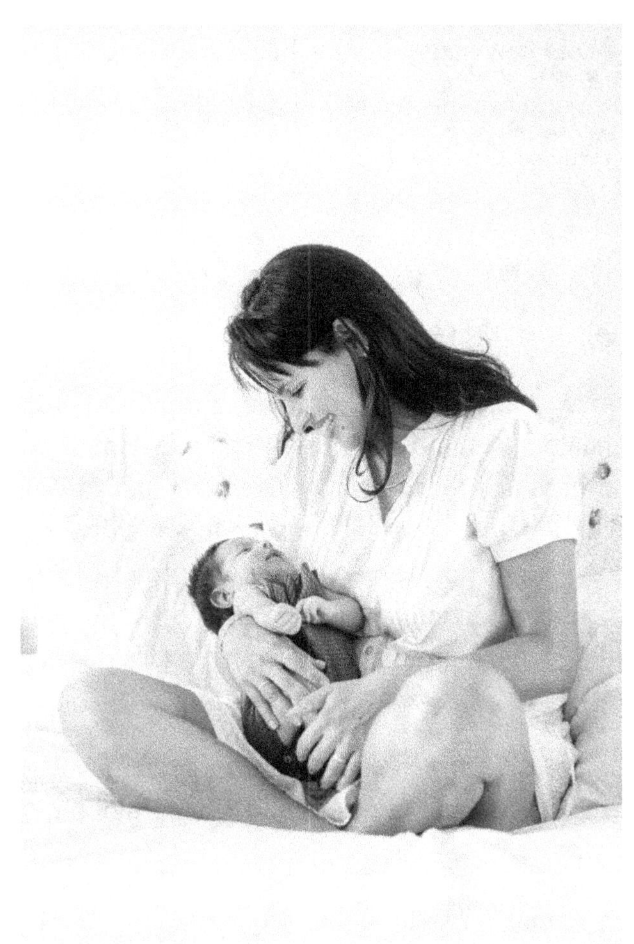

After giving birth, there is a period of adjustment and recuperation. You must keep in mind to look for yourself throughout those first few weeks, whether you gave birth vaginally or by C-section, so that you may recuperate fully. This new stage of your life includes getting plenty of rest, minimizing guests, and creating a routine with your infant.

How you can look after yourself after giving birth

You may believe that after you give birth, you can immediately resume your usual routine. However, this period in your life is full of recuperating and adjusting to life with a baby. It's crucial to keep in mind that delivery requires your body to recuperate over time. Your body needs time to recuperate after any form of delivery, including vaginal birth and cesarean surgery (C-section).

It might sometimes seem daunting to have a newborn infant at home for the first month. Even though it may seem like all of your attention is on taking care of your infant, remember to look after yourself as well. There is some validity to the adage "if you don't take care of yourself, you can't take care of your kid," which you may have heard. After giving birth, there are various things you should keep in mind to look after your health.

Observe the following physical recommendations:

Resting: Giving birth to a child is a laborious job, so, likely, you didn't get much sleep at the hospital. You should take advantage of every opportunity to relax during the crucial first few weeks after giving birth. When your infant is sleeping, try to sleep or relax. You'll be better off after this rest.

Avoiding heavy lifting: While you're healing, stay away from lifting anything heavier than your child. This is particularly crucial if you had a C-section birth.

Washing your hands: It may seem little, but wash your hands often. After using the restroom, after changing your child's diaper, and before feeding them, wash your hands.

Keeping your stair climbing to a minimum: During the first week, you should strive to limit your stair climbing. While you're recovering, try to reduce the number of trips you make up and down stairs each day.

Keeping your baby's care simple: It might be challenging to learn your baby's routine and wants during the first few weeks; don't add more things to your to-do list by worrying about their needs. Your infant does not need a wash each day. Instead, make sure your baby's face, hands, and diaper region are cleansed each day by using wet wipes.

Some social advice to keep in mind is

Limiting visitors: Visitors will want to stop over and say hello to your newest family member. But maybe this isn't the finest moment to play hostess to visitors. Recognize that it's OK to restrict visits or flat-out decline invitations during the first few weeks. You will be mending from your birth and adapting to your new life with your baby throughout this period. You will be creating feeding schedules if you want to breastfeed.

Do not be reluctant to seek assistance: Inform your loved ones and friends of the ways they may assist you. This might be preparing meals, assisting with washing, doing housework, watching after younger siblings, or going to the shop to buy food and supplies.

Do not aim for perfection: Try not to worry about little messes when you do have guests. People are visiting you and your new baby, not your spotless house. During this period, resist the need to make your house seem flawless.

What is postpartum depression after birth, and symptoms you should watch out for

A frequent ailment that affects many new parents is postpartum depression. After giving birth, a complicated combination of physical, mental, and behavioral changes may occur that might make you feel melancholy. The term "baby blues" may also be used to describe a change in some people's emotional state after giving birth. Postpartum depression may include a variety of negative emotions, including sorrow, worry, despair, guilt, and exhaustion.

Contact your healthcare practitioner immediately away if you feel or think any of the following things:

Every day for the last two weeks, I've felt down for most of the day.

Difficulty doing routine household duties for your infant or your self-care.

If your feelings alter after delivery, it's crucial to speak to someone else. It might be challenging to talk to friends, family, or your doctor at times, but you'll usually discover that they want to support you.

How can I maintain my physical health after giving birth?

Once you have a kid, your medical treatment doesn't end. You will still need to set visits with your doctor and take measures to ensure a speedy recovery. You should make an appointment with your obstetrician for a follow-up visit one week following birth. Typically, this is planned to happen four to six weeks following birth. Sometimes, such as two weeks following birth, this appointment may be set up a bit early.

As directed by your healthcare practitioner, you should also take care of your perineum. After giving delivery, you will get comprehensive instructions on how to take care of your perineum. Normally, you'll continue to follow these directions up until your next checkup.

Additional considerations for your postpartum treatment include:

Wait to engage in sexual activity until after your first checkup. After having birth, your body needs time to repair, and delaying sex for a few weeks is a necessary step in that healing. When your perineum has healed (or the abdominal scar from your C-section has healed), and when your postpartum bleeding and discharge are mild, your doctor will advise you that it is safe to have sex again.

Talking about birth control. It may seem unusual to consider becoming pregnant again so soon after giving birth, especially if your period hasn't started up yet. But you most certainly can. Before your child is even born, your doctor will often discuss birth control methods with you. If you haven't already, bring it up with your doctor during your first checkup. You can still get pregnant while nursing even if you aren't menstruating.

Not using tampons or douching during the first several weeks after giving birth. In the first four to six weeks after birth, you shouldn't use a tampon or douche. The safest way to collect blood or discharge is using pads.

Keep taking your daily prenatal vitamins. You may take a multivitamin containing iron if you run out of prenatal vitamins.

Eat nutritious food. Eat a lot of nutritious meals in the weeks after birth. You'll recover faster if you eat well. You should also abstain from coffee and alcohol throughout this period.

Every day, sip from eight huge glasses of water. When attempting to do this, water, juice, and milk are all suitable options.

Go on a stroll. It's beneficial to get out of the home sometimes and get some exercise. After giving birth, walking is a gentle approach to resume exercising. How much exercise you can perform at once and when you may start a new fitness regimen safely should be discussed with your healthcare physician.

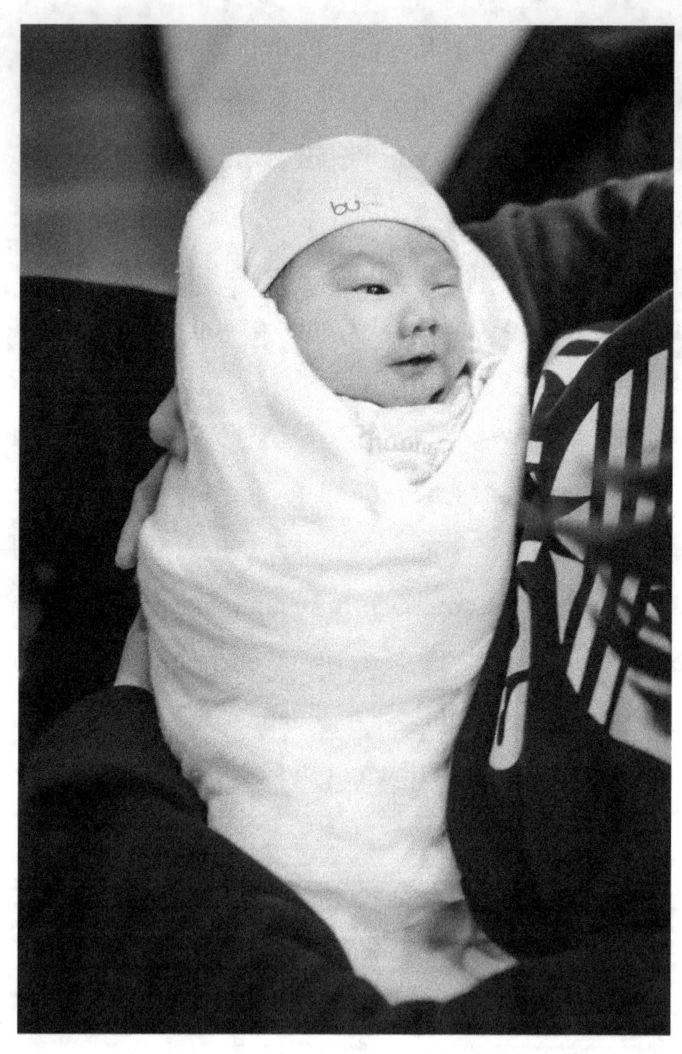

Chapter 9: Caring for your newborn at home

The bulk of your time will be spent feeding, changing diapers, and soothing your infant during the first few weeks of life. At times, you could feel overburdened. Being unsure about your abilities is common, particularly for first-time parents. Every day, it becomes simpler to care for a newborn. Soon, you'll be able to interpret your baby's cries and determine what he or she needs and desires.

The treatment and security of your kid depend heavily on follow-up care. Make careful to schedule and keep all visits, and if your kid has issues, contact your doctor or nurse call line. Additionally, it's a good idea to keep track of your child's medications and test results.

What you are expected to during home care

Feeding. Give your infant food as needed. This implies that you should feed your baby whenever they look hungry, either breastmilk or a bottle. Create no schedule. Your kid will nurse at least eight times per day for the first two weeks. Formula-fed babies may need fewer feedings—at least 6 per day.

These early meals are often brief. A newborn may sometimes merely breastfeed or take a few minutes of bottle feeding. A steady feeding schedule will last longer.

In the first few days after delivery, you may need to rouse your drowsy infant to feed them.

Sleeping

Your infant should never be placed to sleep on their stomach or front. By doing so, the chance of SIDS is decreased (SIDS).

The average newborn sleeps for roughly 18 hours every day. At least once every two to three hours, they briefly awaken.

Babies may experience active sleep. The infant can cry or become agitated. This lasts for a few minutes on average and occurs around every 50 to 60 minutes.

Your infant could first snooze through loud sounds. Your infant can be awakened later by sounds.

Your infant will typically be hungry when they wake up and will need feeding.

Changing diapers and bowel habits

At least every two hours, try to check your baby's diaper. Change it as soon as you can if it has to be modified. That will lessen the chance of diaper rash.

You may learn a lot about your newborn's health by looking at how dirty and wet their diapers are. Babies who are not receiving enough breast milk or formula or who have fluid loss from diarrhea, vomiting, or fever may become dehydrated.

Your infant may need three wet diaper changes every day during the first several days. After that, during the first month of life, anticipate 6 or more wet diapers each day. If you use disposable diapers, it may be challenging to determine whether a diaper is moist. Put a piece of tissue in the diaper if you're unsure. Your infant will pee on it, leaving it moist.

Keep note of your child's typical or regular bowel movements.

Care for umbilical cord

Keep the diaper folded down to the stump on your child.

If that is unsuccessful, you should first cut away a little portion of the diaper's top so that the chord will remain exposed to air.

Instead of washing your child in a tub or sink, sponge bathes them to protect the chord.

The stub ought to disappear in a week or two.

When should you seek assistance?

Dial your baby's doctor right away or get emergency treatment if

The rectal temperature of your infant is 38°C or higher or less than 36.6°C. If you are unable to take your baby's temperature but they seem to be warm, call.

Your infant has gone six hours without a wet diaper.

The skin or eye whites of your newborn get a brighter or deeper yellow.

On or around the stump of the umbilical cord, you see pus or red skin. They are indicators of an infection.

Keep an eye out for any changes in your child's health and call your doctor or nurse right once if you see any of the following:

Based on his or her age, your infant is not experiencing regular bowel movements.

Your infant screams unusually loudly or for an unusually long period.

Your infant sleeps a lot, doesn't wake up for feedings, is fussy, seems to be too exhausted to eat, or doesn't seem to be interested in food.

Bonus 1: 27 Simple method to build bonds with your baby

All of these sweet forms of bonding—which are essential to healthy infant development—include cuddling, playing, and even making goo-goo eyes at your child.

Have you ever noticed how the most Oscar-winning blockbuster can never compare to the beauty of your baby's face, with those chubby cheeks, sparkling eyes, and mischievous smile? It is not a coincidence. It's in your genetic makeup to genuinely enjoy each other's company. And you could prepare your child for a lifetime of wonderful relationships if you trust your gut and establish a strong rapport now.

Feedings create a bond. It's not just about nutrition either, because when your baby cuddles up next to you to nurse or take a bottle, he hears your heartbeat, smells your scent, and feels comforted by skin-to-skin contact.

Send a message to your child. You'll feel like a hero as your child coos and giggles in delight, and the advantages of baby massage are astounding.

Do not use your phone frequently. Currently, if it takes you a few hours to reply to a text, your family, friends, and coworkers will be understanding. Take advantage of the opportunity to spend more time with your child.

Observe each other in the mirror. It's okay if your baby doesn't fully grasp what a reflection is just yet. Baby faces are fascinating to them, so this is a wonderful opportunity to show them your face up close.

Take note of their heartbeat. Do you recall how delighted you were to hear that pleasant sound during sonograms? Now, whenever you want, it can be music to your ears.

Sleep when your child is sleeping. Do not feel bad for going to bed at 7 o'clock, we say. Your baby will gain the most from you as a rested.

Make your partner feel special. Your baby is absorbing the bond between their parents whether you're aware of it or not. Strengthen it by preparing a special meal or setting aside time to watch a movie together, just like in the good old days!

Meet skin-to-skin. Physical connection is essential for a baby's development whether or not you carried your child physically. Being skin-to-skin with a baby is known as kangaroo care, and it's a cute activity that also serves a useful purpose by regulating the baby's breathing and heart rate.

Attend to your infant's cries. Your infant needs to trust you, especially during the first three months of life, and being picked up when they cry fosters that trust. If you decide to sleep-train your child, we assure you that you won't be spoiling them and that the appropriate time will come.

Make swaddling your profession. A baby may sleep better when properly swaddled. More information is not necessary. Utilize this advice.

linger in the glider for a while. Your infant has just fallen asleep, and you're pretty sure you can use your ninja skills to put them in the bassinet without waking them up. But feel free to rock back and forth together in the quiet, dark room before putting them down. Any little thing can lead to a bonding moment!

Dress up for fun. Let's face it; you smile a little when you see your child dressed in a new outfit. If you stage a baby fashion show for your amusement, nobody will judge you!

Journal regularly. Record all the wonderful memories you're creating with your baby because the first year will fly by in a flash. Feel free to find the diary when they invite their first date over to the house in 16 years!

Have a meet and greet with a plush animal. You'll love seeing your child interact with their furry friends by touching, smelling, and even tasting them. Pay attention as they choose a favorite; you'll want to have that book available at bedtime.

To your child, read aloud. It's never too early to encourage your child's inner reader! If you can give each character a distinct voice, you will receive bonus points.

While your baby is crying remember to breathe. Every baby cries; the mother at Pilates who looks flawlessly put together and claims her child never cries is lying. Your baby will scream more if you become tense or angry, though. Remind yourself that even grownups get upset; babies simply lack the language to do so.

Plan your time. Babies are creatures of routine, so if you follow a routine, your child will feel more at ease. As you anticipate their feeding needs, it will also help your baby realize that you are the one performing all the magic.

Go on a date with your Child. Are you feeling Adventure? Go to the zoo! Not a daredevil? Around the corner is a working coffee shop. Leaving your tiny cocoon with the infant will serve as a reminder that the world is still spinning.

Decide on a pet name. You may call your child anything you want since you are the parent. The nickname you choose will also function as private communication between the two of you.

Organize a playlist. Choose five of your favorite songs, play them often for the infant, and join in as you sing. When they ultimately start to hop along, you'll enjoy it immensely, and it's always beneficial for your baby to hear your voice.

Bring out the old family portraits. Perhaps your kid will inherit your grin, eyes, or ringlets. You'll feel an immediate connection to any similarity you discover.

Enjoy the feeding time. Do not be concerned about the mess when it is time to introduce solids (about 6 months). Instead, pay attention to the delightful delight and exploration of the novel tastes, textures, and fragrances your baby is experiencing.

Take a funny stance. Have a great time wriggling your eyebrows and sticking out your tongue, and be ready for your heart to melt when you eventually get your baby to grin.

Are you anxious? Talk with your child. Feel free to share your feelings with your new tiny BFF since those first few months of parenting might be lonely. Most likely, they will enjoy hearing your voice, and you'll feel like a burden has been removed. Do you hear "win/win"?

Make fun of the crap. We said it, after all. The act of changing a baby's diaper is sometimes considered unpleasant, but you may make it enjoyable by humming a cheerful tune while you wipe, ogling your baby's adorable bottom, or thinking up a million new terms for excrement.

Smooch those adorable tiny lips. Your kid may very likely wipe off your kisses and give you "that look" in a few years, but now? So pucker up, they are so cutely helpless.

week by week First time mom needs for Taking Care

BONUS 2

Weekly Pregnancy Belly measurements

Weeks	Measurements	Feeling
Week 1		
Week 2		
Week 3		
Week 4		
Week 5		
Week 6		
Week 7		
Week 8		
Week 9		
Week 10		
Week 11		

Week 12		
Week 13		
Week 14		
Week 15		
Week 16		
Week 17		
Week 18		
Week 19		

Week 20		
Week 21		
Week 22		
Week 23		

Week 24		
Week 25		
Week 26		
Week 27		
Week 28		
Week 29		
Week 30		
Week 31		
Week 32		
Week 33		
Week 34		
Week 35		
Week 36		

Week 37		
Week38		
Week39		
Week 40		

Weekly Pregnancy weight tracker

Weeks	Weight
Week 1	
Week 2	
Week 3	
Week 4	
Week 5	
Week 6	
Week 7	
Week 8	
Week 9	
Week 10	
Week 11	
Week 12	
Week 13	
Week	

14	
Week 15	
Week 16	
Week 17	
Week 18	
Week 19	

Week 20	
Week 21	
Week 22	
Week 23	
Week 24	
Week 25	
Week 26	
Week 27	

Week 28	
Week 29	
Week 30	
Week 31	
Week 32	
Week 33	
Week 34	
Week 35	
Week 36	

Week 37	
Week 38	
Week 39	
Week 40	

Weekly Prenatal vitamin tracker

Weeks	Mon	Tue	Wed	Thu	Fri	Sat	Sun
1							
2							
3							
4							
5							
6							
7							
8							
9							
10							
11							
12							

Weeks	Mon	Tue	Wed	Thu	Fri	Sat	Sun

13							
14							
15							
16							
17							
18							
19							
20							
21							
22							
23							
24							

Weeks	Mon	Tue	Wed	Thu	Fri	Sat	Sun
25							
26							
27							
28							

29							
30							
31							
32							
33							
34							
35							
36							

Weeks	Mon	Tue	Wed	Thu	Fri	Sat	Sun
37							
38							
39							
40							